21ST CENTURY SCHIZOID HEALTH CARE

ALSO BY ARTHUR LAZARUS

Neuroleptic Malignant Syndrome and Related Conditions (co-author)

Controversies in Managed Mental Health Care

Career Pathways in Psychiatry: Transition in Changing Times

MD/MBA: Physicians on the New Frontier of Medical Management

Every Story Counts: Exploring Contemporary Practice Through Narrative Medicine

Medicine on Fire: A Narrative Travelogue

Narrative Medicine: The Fifth Vital Sign

Narrative Medicine: Harnessing the Power of Storytelling through Essays

Story Treasures: Medical Essays and Insights in the Narrative Tradition

21st Century Schizoid Health Care

Essays and Reflections to Keep You Sane
on Your Medical Travels

Arthur Lazarus, MD, MBA

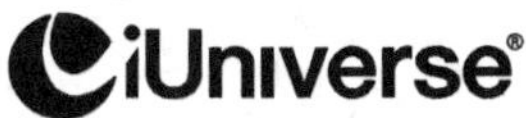

21st CENTURY SCHIZOID HEALTH CARE
ESSAYS AND REFLECTIONS TO KEEP YOU SANE ON YOUR MEDICAL TRAVELS

iUniverse books may be ordered through booksellers or by contacting:

iUniverse
1663 Liberty Drive
Bloomington, IN 47403
www.iuniverse.com
844-349-9409

ISBN: 978-1-6632-6768-9 (sc)
ISBN: 978-1-6632-6769-6 (e)

Library of Congress Control Number: 2024921226

Print information available on the last page.

iUniverse rev. date: 10/10/2024

To Nolan, Norah, Noam, Layla, and Owen,
May your generation lead us toward a healthier, saner future.

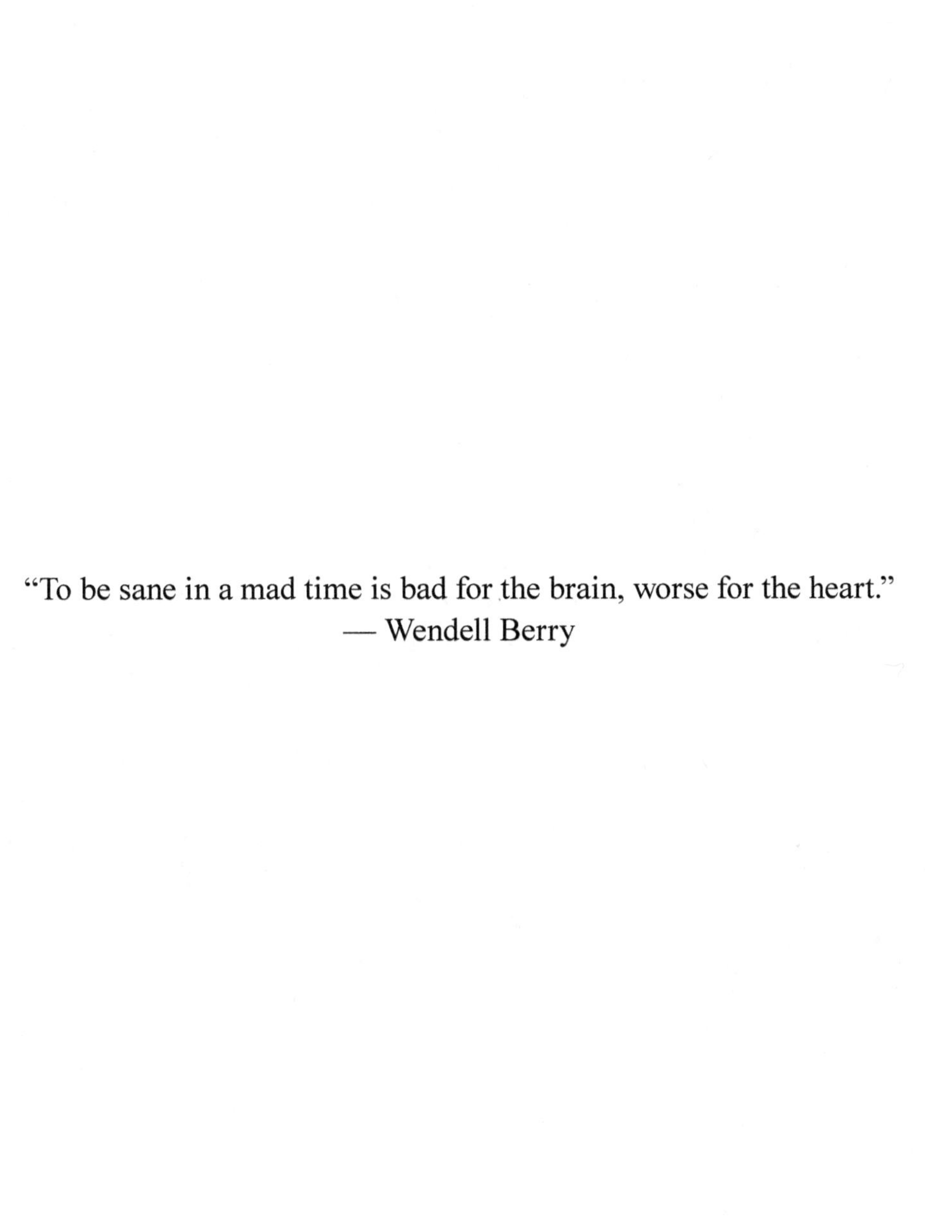

"To be sane in a mad time is bad for the brain, worse for the heart."
— Wendell Berry

Contents

Reflections

Afterword

Preface

In the past few years, both during and after the coronavirus pandemic, I have reflected on countless stories of everyday hope and despair. With more free time than usual, my son suggested, "Why don't you write your autobiography?" Taking his advice, I decided to write essays and op-eds about the hidden crisis in American medicine rather than pen a traditional autobiography. This endeavor resulted in a series of books that entwine memoirs from my career as a psychiatrist. This book is the sixth installment in that series.

Within these pages, I delve into provocative and controversial topics in health care, interlacing stories from my career and personal life experiences. The narratives exude a sense of restrained optimism amid the pain and loss tied to illness and suffering. An acute awareness of mortality and life's fragility has deeply influenced me, and these essays stem from those sentiments, often presenting critical viewpoints on health care.

My main objective was to provide readers with an insight into American medicine, contemplating both its historical context and the changing landscape. In an age where information is abundant yet often overwhelming, where technological advances coexist with persistent health disparities, and where mental and physical well-being are increasingly recognized as deeply interconnected yet remain functionally separate, maintaining a coherent and balanced approach to health can seem like an elusive goal.

This book was intended to provide a beacon through the fog, offering clarity, wisdom, and a touch of humor to help readers stay grounded and informed on their medical journeys. My essays and reflections aim to resonate with healthcare professionals and anyone seeking a better understanding of their own health and the inner workings of the U.S. healthcare system, where an estimated 80% of physicians are now employed by hospitals, health systems, and corporations, and small independent practices are rapidly vanishing.

Within this sea change, the path to well-being remains deeply personal and unique. Yet, it is essential that we are still able to share common challenges and triumphs along the way. It is my hope that these narratives will not only provide valuable, uplifting insights, but also foster a sense of community and shared experience. In a world that can often feel disjointed and "schizoid," may these essays serve as a guide to help readers navigate with greater ease and confidence.

Thank you for embarking on this journey with me. Here's to staying healthy, sane, and whole in the 21st century.

PROLOGUE

1. 21st Century Schizoid Health Care

The U.S. system is broken and possibly beyond repair.

"21st Century Schizoid Man" is a 1969 antiwar song by the progressive ("prog") rock band King Crimson. It appears as the lead cut on their debut album *In the Court of the Crimson King.* "Schizoid Man" is considered an epic, described by *Rolling Stone* as "a seven-and-a-half-minute statement of purpose: rock power, jazz spontaneity, and classical precision harnessed in the service of a common aim."

While recently listening to "Schizoid Man" for the umpteenth time, it dawned on me that "schizoid" and its many synonyms – fractured, fragmented, splintered, and so on – is an appropriate way to characterize the U.S. healthcare system. *Schizo* is a Latinized version of a Greek word meaning "split." "Schizoid" aptly describes the way health care is delivered and experienced today: disconnected and impersonal. For sure, the system is broken.

Just as a schizoid individual might struggle to integrate different aspects of their personality, the U.S. health care system struggles to deliver services in a coherent fashion. Patients often have to navigate a complex web of providers, insurers, and healthcare facilities, leading to gaps in care and communication breakdowns (think Led Zeppelin here). This fragmentation can result in patients receiving inconsistent information and care, complicating their course of treatment and potentially leading to poorer health outcomes.

The American health system lacks clear goals and suffers from inconsistent policies at federal, state, and local levels. It invokes the directionless thinking I observed in individuals with schizoid personality disorder. Inconsistencies lead to confusion and inefficiency, with patients receiving different levels of care and coverage based on their location or insurance provider. These policy discrepancies create a landscape where accessing healthcare services is challenging, further exacerbating the system's dysfunction.

Moreover, there are significant disparities in accessing quality health care, similar to how a schizoid individual might struggle to form consistent and meaningful connections. These disparities can be based on socioeconomic status, race, and geographic location, leading to unequal health outcomes. Such inequities highlight the system's inability to provide uniform care across diverse populations, undermining public health efforts and social equity.

Patients often experience the health care system as soulless, akin to the way people with schizoid personality disorder usually appear: emotionally detached. This can lead to feelings of alienation and frustration, further complicating the doctor-patient relationship and overall satisfaction with care. The lack of personalized, compassionate interactions can diminish trust in the system and deter individuals from seeking necessary medical attention.

The economic aspects of the U.S. healthcare system can be seen as schizoid insofar as the cost of care and the value received are disconnected. Patients often face exorbitant, surprise medical bills, while the system as a whole struggles with inefficiencies and waste. This economic dysfunction reflects a lack of coherence in how health care is financed and delivered, burdening individuals and families with financial strain and complicating the overall sustainability of healthcare provision.

The truth is, the U.S. does not have a health care system; it has a revenue generating system that does health care. In it, income takes precedence over patient outcomes. Private equity (PE) firms are silently completing the "financialization" of health care, having invested nearly $1 trillion in approximately 8,000 health care deals over the past decade. PE companies pool money from investors to acquire hospitals, physicians' practices, nursing homes, mental health facilities, home care services, hospices, and ambulance services. They build them into bigger enterprises, and then sell them. In doing so, they suck the resources out of America's medical enterprises, and feed on doctors to generate profits for the PE owners.

Rather than being a social good, health care has now become a series of market driven financial transactions where PE-owning healthcare services is not the disease but rather the symptom of health care being viewed as a commodity. As a result, patients are more likely to experience adverse health events, like infections or falls, at PE-owned hospitals, according to a 2023 *JAMA* study. Other research has linked PE ownership to higher costs for patients and payers, and some studies have found harmful impacts to healthcare quality in nursing homes. Quite simply, PE is ravaging U.S. health care.

Leaders in medicine are aware of this very disturbing trend, but they lack significant financial enforcement capabilities, or the legislative power, to institute needed changes including the push for greater transparency and for exposing deceptive practices of PE. Political divisions, vested interests, and varying ideologies contribute to a lack of cohesive strategy for improving the system, resulting in piecemeal solutions that fail to address the root problems. This persistent inability to enact comprehensive reform underscores the systemic issues that hinder effective, equitable, and efficient health care delivery.

But as my colleague and population health expert David Nash, MD, MBA, has repeatedly emphasized, we know how to fix what's broken in the U.S. healthcare system. Nash and associates have described the characteristics of an optimal healthcare model – and it does not entail any new "aha!" observations. In terms of model design, the components include:

- Transitioning from system-centered to person-centered orientation

- Considering the "whole person" over a lifetime
- Shifting from sick care to health care
- Making healthcare equitable and easy to access and use for all persons
- Taking a long-term perspective on relationships and investments (e.g., optimization of outcomes that people value, investment in sustainability and well-being of the workforce, capabilities for anticipating, responding, and adapting to public health crises)
- Fostering a culture of continuous improvement
- Increasing the value of current spending before seeking to reduce costs

The hard part, according to Nash, is "building and promoting a new model that will succeed where so many other well-intended and carefully constructed models have failed (or inadvertently created more problems)." Nash admits he is familiar with the Herculean effort required to implement even a small change in a single sphere, and he has many doubts. So do I.

Perhaps it's time for universal health care. A 2024 *Commonwealth Fund* report compared health system performance in 10 countries and concluded: "The U.S. continues to be in a class by itself in the underperformance of its health care sector. While the other nine countries differ in the details of their systems and in their performance on domains, unlike the U.S., they all have found a way to meet their residents' most basic health care needs, *including universal coverage* [italics added]."

When King Crimson wrote "21st Century Schizoid Man," they couldn't have possibly foreshadowed the broken U.S. healthcare system as it exists today, not least because they were a British band. Still, the song's heavily distorted vocals are reminiscent of patients' perceptions of their healthcare journey, likewise distorted, making it difficult for them to feel that their care is genuinely respected and well-managed. Interfacing with the medical system has become demoralizing and degrading – and the overall prognosis seems no better than that for an individual diagnosed with schizoid personality disorder: poor, at best.

ESSAYS

2. Prophecy and Prognostication – Part 1

"The wall on which the prophets wrote is cracking at the seams."
—Words and music by King Crimson, from "Epitaph"

Virtually every patient, when first diagnosed with a serious disorder, wants to know their prognosis. The word "prognosis" comes from the Greek "prognōsis," which means "foreknowledge" or "foresight." In the medical field, a prognosis refers to the likely course and outcome of a disease or medical condition, essentially predicting how the patient's health will progress.

Similarly, "prophecy" comes from the Greek "prophēteia," meaning "the gift of interpreting the will of the gods" or "foretelling." Prophecy traditionally involves predicting future events, often with a divine or supernatural element.

While a prognosis represents a specific, scientific prediction related to health and disease outcomes, prophecy encompasses a broader and often spiritual or mystical prediction of future events, Both involve an element of foresight and prediction, but they differ significantly in context and application.

The concept of prophecy and the role of prophets have deep roots in human history, spanning various cultures and religions. Prophecy, in its essence, is the act of conveying messages or insights believed to be divinely inspired, often concerning future events or hidden knowledge. Prophets, therefore, are individuals regarded as intermediaries who convey these divine messages to the people.

One of the earliest known instances of prophecy can be traced back to ancient Mesopotamia, where prophets were often associated with temples and played a crucial role in interpreting the will of the gods. They used various methods, including divination and interpreting omens, to make predictions. Similarly, in ancient Egypt, prophecy was closely linked to the priesthood and the interpretation of dreams. Pharaohs often consulted prophets or seers for guidance on state affairs and military campaigns.

The Hebrew Bible (Old Testament) provides a rich tapestry of prophetic tradition. Prophets like Isaiah, Jeremiah, and Ezekiel were central figures who spoke on behalf of Yahweh, addressing moral, social, and political issues. Their prophecies often included calls for repentance and warnings of divine judgment. In classical antiquity, the Greeks had their own tradition of prophecy, exemplified by the Oracle of Delphi. The Pythia, or priestess, would deliver cryptic messages believed to be inspired by the god Apollo. Similarly, Roman prophets, or augurs, interpreted the will of the gods through the observation of natural phenomena, such as the flight patterns of birds.

In Islam, prophets (nabi) and messengers (rasul) are fundamental to the faith. Muhammad is considered the final prophet, delivering the ultimate guidance through the Quran. Other prophets in Islam include figures also recognized in Judaism and Christianity, such as Moses (Musa), Abraham (Ibrahim), and Jesus (Isa).

The intersection of prophecy and medicine is a fascinating aspect of history, particularly in how ancient societies understood health and disease. In many ancient cultures, the roles of healer and prophet were often intertwined. Shamans, medicine men, and other traditional healers were believed to possess both medical knowledge and the ability to communicate with the spiritual realm. They would often use rituals, divination, and herbal remedies to heal the sick, guided by prophetic insights.

In ancient Greece, the god Asclepius was associated with healing and prophecy. The serpent-entwined rod (staff) of Asclepius is the traditional symbol of medicine. The Asclepian temples, or Asclepieia, served as centers for both medical treatment and prophetic dreams.

Patients would undergo incubation, a process of sleeping in the temple to receive divine messages about their ailments and cures.

During the medieval period, the influence of religious prophecy on medicine was significant. Monastic hospitals and Islamic medical institutions often combined spiritual care with medical treatment. The Renaissance saw a revival of interest in ancient texts, including those that blended medicine with astrology and alchemy. Figures like Paracelsus, a Swiss physician, and alchemist, believed in the interconnectedness of the spiritual and physical realms, incorporating elements of prophecy into his medical practice.

A notable figure during the Renaissance was Nostradamus, a French physician, and seer. His prophecies, a collection of 942 poetic quatrains, have intrigued and puzzled scholars and the public for centuries. Nostradamus's background in medicine and his reputed ability to foresee future events highlight the enduring connection between healing and prophetic insight during this period.

In contemporary medicine, the role of prophecy has largely been supplanted by scientific inquiry and evidence-based practice. However, the historical influence of prophetic traditions can still be seen in holistic and alternative medicine practices that emphasize the mind-body-spirit connection. Although Hippocrates distanced his practice from the supernatural, emphasizing natural causes and empirical observation, the tradition of seeking divine guidance in medicine has persisted alongside more rational approaches. It is not uncommon to hear someone utter "thank God" when given good medical news.

Prognosis has become a key aspect of the physician's role, relying on observation, experience, and increasingly, scientific evidence. Physicians are often seen as having a prophetic role when delivering a prognosis, especially in cases of terminal illness. The weight of predicting a patient's future, especially when it involves life or death, carries a gravity reminiscent of the ancient prophets' role. The credibility of both prophets and physicians is often linked to the perceived accuracy of their predictions, and their role is both revered and feared in society.

The expectation that physicians can foresee outcomes, despite the inherent limitations in medicine, mirrors the ancient demand for prophetic certainty. This dual legacy of prophecy and prognosis highlights the enduring human desire to understand and predict the future, whether through divine insight or scientific reasoning.

3. Prophecy and Prognostication – Part 2

"The words of the prophets are written on the subway walls and tenement halls."
—Paul Simon, from "The Sound of Silence"

In the 21st century, the development of predictive analytics in medicine represents the latest evolution in the ancient human endeavor of the prophets. Predictive analytics involves using data, statistical algorithms, and machine learning techniques to identify the likelihood of future outcomes based on historical data. In health care, this means leveraging vast amounts of patient data to predict disease onset, progression, and treatment outcomes. This modern form of prognosis is far removed from the mystical origins of prophecy, yet it fulfills a similar role: offering insight into the future to guide decision-making and prognostication.

Predictive analytics has revolutionized many aspects of medicine. For example, it is now possible to predict the likelihood of a patient developing certain conditions, such as diabetes or cardiovascular disease, based on genetic markers, lifestyle factors, and previous medical history. This allows for earlier intervention and personalized treatment plans, which can significantly improve patient outcomes. Similarly, predictive models can estimate the risk of complications during surgery or the likelihood of a patient's readmission to the hospital, enabling more precise and proactive care.

The integration of artificial intelligence (AI) further enhances predictive capabilities (see essay 8). Machine learning algorithms can continuously learn and adapt from new data, refining predictions and providing deeper insights. AI-powered tools can analyze medical images, detect anomalies, and even predict disease progression based on subtle patterns that may elude human observation.

However, the rise of predictive analytics also raises important ethical and practical questions, reminiscent of those faced by ancient prophets. Just as prophets were held accountable for the accuracy of their predictions, modern physicians and data scientists must grapple with the limitations and potential biases of predictive models. The accuracy of these models depends on the quality and diversity of the data they are trained on. Inaccuracies can lead to misdiagnosis, inappropriate treatment, or inequities in health care. Moreover, the growing reliance on predictive analytics may reduce the role of human judgment in medicine, as algorithms increasingly guide decisions that were once the sole domain of physicians.

Furthermore, just as prophecies could influence behavior by shaping expectations about the future, predictive analytics can also have a self-fulfilling effect. For instance, a prediction that a patient is at high risk for a particular condition might lead to more intensive monitoring or intervention, which could, in turn, effect the course of the disease ("Hawthorne effect"). This intertwining of prediction and outcome complicates the ethical landscape, as the line between foresight and causation becomes blurred.

Paul Simon's line, "the words of the prophets are written on the subway walls and tenement halls" suggests that the profound truths and insights once delivered by prophets are now found in the everyday graffiti and messages scrawled in urban environments. "The Sound of Silence" as a whole addresses themes of alienation and the lack of real communication in modern society, including medicine (see essay 21). The evocative imagery of the song can be used to convey a sense of lost wisdom replaced by computer intelligence, and the need to pay attention to the voices and messages that emerge from the heart as well as the brain.

Despite these concerns, the future of prognostication in medicine seems bright. The interplay between prophecy, prognosis, and predictive analytics promises to revolutionize health care. The integration of AI, big data, and personalized medicine will continue to enhance our ability to foresee medical outcomes and tailor treatments to individual patients. This evolution represents a natural extension of the ancient art of prophecy, now grounded in scientific rigor and technological innovation.

The journey from prophecy to prognosis to predictive analytics reflects humanity's preoccupation with the future. Each stage in this evolution – from the mystical insights of ancient prophets to the empirical predictions of early physicians to the data-driven forecasts of modern medicine – has brought us closer to realizing forthcoming events. Yet, with each advance comes new challenges and responsibilities.

As we continue to refine our ability to predict medical outcomes, we must remain mindful of the ethical implications and ensure that these tools are used to enhance, rather than diminish, the human element of health care. While the methods have evolved, the underlying goal remains the same: to provide treatment guidance, alleviate suffering, and promote well-being. As we embrace the future of medicine, the legacy of prophecy lives on, enriched by the power of data and the promise of predictive insights.

4. Finding Balance Between Burnout and Longevity

Approximately half of physicians in the U.S. report at least one symptom of burnout.

In Neil Young's song "My My, Hey Hey (Out of the Blue)" he wrote, "It's better to burn out than to fade away." John Lennon responded, "It's better to fade away like an old soldier than to burn out."

Here is the complete transcript of Lennon talking to David Sheff, who interviewed Lennon in September 1980 for *Playboy* magazine (reprinted in the book *The Playboy Interviews with John Lennon and Yoko Ono*):

"If he [Young] was talking about burning out like Sid Vicious, forget it. I don't appreciate the worship of dead Sid Vicious or of dead James Dean or dead John Wayne. It's the same thing. Making Sid Vicious a hero, Jim Morrison – it's garbage to me. I worship the people who survive – Gloria Swanson, Greta Garbo. They're saying John Wayne conquered cancer – he whipped it like a man. You know, I'm sorry that he died and all that – I'm sorry for his family – but he didn't whip cancer. It whipped him. I don't want Sean [Lennon's son with Yoko Ono] worshiping John Wayne or Johnny Rotten or Sid Vicious. What do they teach you? Nothing. Death. Sid Vicious died for what? So that we might rock? I mean, it's garbage you know. If Neil Young admires that sentiment so much, why doesn't he do it? Because he sure as hell faded away and came back many times, like all of us. No, thank you. I'll take the living and the healthy."

Young replied to Lennon when the former was interviewed by Cameron Crowe (in *Musician,* November 1982). Lennon had already been dead two years. Young told Crowe:

"The rock 'n' roll spirit is not survival. Of course, the people who play rock 'n' roll should survive. But the essence of the rock 'n' roll spirit, to me, is that it's better to burn out really bright than it is to sort of decay off into infinity. Even though if you look at it in a mature way, you think, well yes...you should decay off into infinity, and keep going along. Rock 'n' roll doesn't look that far ahead. Rock 'n' roll is right now. What's happening right this second. Is it bright? Or is it dim because it's waiting for tomorrow – that's what people want to know. That's why I say that."

Neil Young and John Lennon reflect different perspectives on life and legacy, which can also be applied metaphorically to the practice of medicine. Is there a clear choice between these two extremes of philosophy? In the medical field, the balance between "burning out" and "fading away" can be interpreted in various ways, particularly in terms of career longevity, work-life balance, and the quality of care provided to patients.

A physician who "burns out" might be seen as someone who works intensely and passionately, potentially making significant contributions in a short period. This could lead to breakthroughs, innovations, or highly impactful patient care. However, the downside of this approach is the risk of physical and emotional exhaustion, which can lead to professional burnout. This not only affects the physician's health and well-being but can also compromise patient safety and the quality of care.

Conversely, a physician who "fades away" might be someone who maintains a steady, sustainable pace over a long career. This approach can lead to a balanced life, long-term professional satisfaction, and consistent patient care. Yet, the potential downside could be a lack of urgency or drive, possibly leading to complacency or a slower rate of innovation and improvement in practice.

A balanced medical approach is often considered ideal. This involves maintaining a manageable workload to prevent burnout while still being productive and impactful, engaging in lifelong learning to stay updated with medical advancements, ensuring that the physician remains effective and innovative. Prioritizing personal well-being and family time to maintain overall life satisfaction and prevent professional fatigue is also crucial. Ensuring that patient care remains the top priority, with a focus on providing high-quality, compassionate, and effective treatment, is essential.

However, achieving balance has proved difficult. In 2023, approximately half of U.S. physicians reported experiencing at least one symptom of burnout, according to the American Medical Association (AMA). Although this percentage fell from 53% in 2022, the AMA noted six specialties that continue to report high rates of burnout:

- Emergency medicine: 56.5%
- Internal medicine: 51.4%
- Ob/gyn: 51.2%
- Family medicine: 51%
- Pediatrics: 46.9%
- Hospital medicine: 44%

Notably, plastic surgery and ophthalmology, with flexibility of practice, customizable hours, few administrative responsibilities, and some of the best compensation of any physician specialties, were the least prone to burnout, with only 37% and 39% of physicians, respectively, experiencing any symptoms.

The AMA report also revealed that more than a quarter of physicians' stress was due to a shortage of physicians and support staff, and 12.7% said their stress was due to the volume of administrative tasks. Thus, while declining rates of burnout are a milestone in efforts to address this epidemic, more work must be done to address the root causes and provide support to physicians in all specialties.

In the final analysis, physicians should not be duped into thinking there is only a choice between burning out or fading away – it is a false dichotomy. They should realize there is a middle ground and strive to maintain a balanced and sustainable career that prioritizes both personal well-being and high-quality patient care, continuously seeking opportunities for professional growth, self-care, and meaningful connections with colleagues, patients, and family.

5. The Role of Influencers in Modern Medicine

Influencers are an important extension to the public and healthcare community.

Being an influencer in today's digital age generally refers to an individual who has the power to affect the purchasing decisions of others because of their authority, knowledge, position, or relationship with their audience. Influencers typically have a dedicated following on social media platforms, where they share content that engages their audience and drives trends. They leverage their reach to promote products, ideas, or behaviors, often collaborating with brands or organizations to enhance their visibility and impact. The role of an influencer transcends mere popularity; it involves a strategic blend of authenticity, consistency, and engagement to build trust and credibility with their followers.

Most influencers originate in the entertainment and sports industries but really any profession is possible. Experts in fields like science, education, technology, and even niche hobbies can also become influential by sharing their knowledge and passion with a wider audience. With the rise of social media and online platforms, anyone with valuable insights or engaging content can build a following and make an impact in their respective fields.

I am reluctant to name key influencers because their popularity fluctuates constantly, much like a revolving door. Social media is highly trend-driven, and influencers who capture the zeitgeist can quickly be in vogue, but as trends shift, new influencers emerge while others drift out to sea. Different social media platforms rise and fall in popularity, and influencers who thrive on a particular platform may struggle if it loses users or changes its algorithms, while others adept at newer platforms can quickly gain prominence.

Public perception of influencers can change rapidly due to scandals, controversies, or changes in personal behavior, leading to a loss of followers and influence, and allowing others to take their place. Audiences can be fickle, constantly seeking fresh content and new perspectives, leading to a continuous cycle of discovering and following new influencers. The market becomes saturated as more people attempt to become influencers, increasing competition and making it harder for any one influencer to maintain long-term dominance. The pressure to constantly produce engaging content can lead to fatigue, causing influencers to take breaks, reduce their online presence, or even leave the industry, making room for new faces.

In the realm of medicine, the concept of an influencer takes on a more nuanced and significant role. Medical influencers are often healthcare professionals, such as doctors, nurses, researchers, or public health experts, who utilize their expertise and platforms to educate, inform, and inspire both their peers and the general public. Their influence is rooted in their professional credentials and evidence-based knowledge, which they use to disseminate accurate health information, debunk myths, and advocate for public health initiatives. These influencers play a crucial role in shaping public perceptions of health and medicine, promoting healthy behaviors, and encouraging adherence to medical guidelines. They may also collaborate with healthcare organizations, participate in public health campaigns, and contribute to policy discussions, thereby extending their influence beyond social media to real-world health outcomes.

Medical influencers can carry considerable weight, particularly in an era where misinformation can spread rapidly online. By providing reliable information and engaging with their audience in a transparent and accessible manner, medical influencers help bridge the gap between complex medical knowledge and the lay public. They can demystify medical procedures, explain the importance of vaccinations, and offer support for mental health issues, among other contributions. Additionally, they often serve as role models within the healthcare community, inspiring other professionals to embrace digital platforms as tools for education and advocacy.

Ultimately, being an influencer in medicine is about leveraging one's expertise and platform to foster a well-informed public, promote health literacy, and contribute to the betterment of society. It requires a commitment to ethical standards, ongoing education, and a genuine passion for improving health outcomes. As the digital landscape continues to evolve, the role of medical influencers will likely become even more integral in shaping the future of healthcare communication and public health efforts.

One prominent example of a medical influencer is Mikhail Varshavski, DO, a board-certified family medicine physician widely known as "Doctor Mike." With more than 12 million followers on platforms like YouTube and Instagram, Dr. Mike uses his platform to discuss a wide range of health topics, from common medical myths to lifestyle tips and the latest medical research. His engaging and personable approach makes complex medical information relatable and easy to understand for a broad audience. Dr. Mike's influence extends beyond social media; he has appeared on numerous television shows and collaborates with health organizations to promote public health initiatives, making him a significant figure in the realm of medical influence.

Another influential figure in medicine is Sanjay Gupta, MD, a practicing neurosurgeon and the chief medical correspondent for CNN. Dr. Gupta's extensive work in journalism allows him to reach a global audience with in-depth reporting on medical and health-related issues. His credibility as a medical professional, combined with his ability to explain intricate medical topics in a clear and concise manner, has earned him the trust of millions. Dr. Gupta's influence is particularly notable during public health crises. During the COVID-19 pandemic, his insights and analyses were vital in guiding public understanding and response.

Nurses also play a crucial role as medical influencers. Nurse Blake, for example, has built a substantial following through his humorous and insightful content that highlights the realities of nursing. By blending humor with education, Nurse Blake addresses serious topics such as mental health, LGBTQ+ awareness, patient care, and the challenges faced by healthcare workers. His content not only entertains but also fosters a sense of community and support among healthcare professionals, while educating the public about the dynamic role nurses play in the healthcare system. Nurse Blake is also a touring comedian, having performed over 200 comedy shows for an audience of over 250,000 nurses worldwide.

Researchers and scientists like Anthony Fauci, MD, the former director of the National Institute of Allergy and Infectious Diseases, also serve as influential figures in medicine. Throughout his career, Dr. Fauci has been a key voice in public health, particularly during the HIV/AIDS epidemic and the COVID-19 pandemic. His extensive knowledge, experience, and calm demeanor have made him a trusted source of information for both the public and policymakers. Dr. Fauci's ability to communicate the importance of scientific research and public health measures has had a positive impact on public health policy and awareness. He advised two Presidents through the COVID-19 pandemic.

Influencers in medicine, ranging from physicians and nurses to researchers and public health experts, play an essential role in modern healthcare communication. Their ability to translate complex medical information into accessible and engaging content helps to educate the public, dispel myths, and promote healthy behaviors. As the digital landscape continues to evolve, the influence of these medical professionals will likely grow, further enhancing their ability to contribute to public health and medical education.

6. Key Opinion Leaders in the Pharmaceutical Industry

Influencers representing "pharma" walk a fine line between promotion and education.

In the pharmaceutical industry, medical influencers are referred to as "key opinion leaders" (KOLs) or "key thought leaders." They play an essential role in bridging the gap between medical research and clinical practice. These influencers, often esteemed healthcare professionals or researchers, rise in prominence due to their expertise, extensive experience, and contributions to medical science. Their opinions and endorsements are highly valued by peers, practitioners, and the industry, making them influential figures in shaping medical practices and the adoption of new therapies.

KOLs typically gain prominence through a combination of academic achievements, clinical expertise, and active participation in medical communities. Many KOLs are authors of influential research papers, speakers at major medical conferences, and leaders of clinical trials. Their visibility in these arenas, combined with their extensive publication records, helps establish their credibility and authority. Additionally, their affiliations with prestigious institutions and their roles in professional societies further enhance their reputations, making them trusted sources of information and guidance within their specialties.

The influence of KOLs on practitioners is multifaceted. Their expertise provides practitioners with insights into the latest advancements in medical science and treatment protocols. KOLs often serve as educators, offering training sessions, workshops, and continuing medical education (CME) courses that help practitioners stay updated with current best practices. Their endorsement of specific therapies or medications can significantly impact prescribing behaviors, as practitioners often look to KOLs for guidance on complex clinical decisions. Moreover, KOLs' involvement in clinical trials and their firsthand experience with new treatments provide valuable real-world evidence that can inform clinical practice.

Pharmaceutical companies recognize the value of KOLs and often collaborate with them to enhance the integrity and reach of their products. KOLs may participate in advisory boards, consult on clinical trial designs, and contribute to the development of educational materials. These collaborations benefit the industry by providing scientific validation and helping to communicate the efficacy and safety of new therapies to the medical community. The endorsement of a respected KOL can accelerate the acceptance and adoption of new treatments, ultimately benefiting patient care.

However, the relationship between KOLs and the pharmaceutical industry raises several ethical issues. One primary concern is the potential for conflicts of interest. Financial relationships between KOLs and pharmaceutical companies can create biases, consciously or unconsciously influencing the KOLs' opinions and recommendations. Transparency is essential in mitigating these concerns; KOLs and companies must disclose any financial ties to ensure that their interactions are conducted ethically and that the information provided to practitioners is trustworthy.

Furthermore, the influence of KOLs must be managed to prevent the undue promotion of off-label (unapproved) uses of medications. While KOLs may have valuable insights into novel applications of therapies, promoting off-label uses without sufficient evidence can pose risks to patient safety. Regulatory bodies and professional societies must provide clear guidelines to ensure that KOLs' communications adhere to ethical standards and prioritize patient welfare.

Another ethical challenge is achieving a balance between education and marketing and recognizing the difference between the two.

While KOLs play a vital role in educating practitioners, there is a risk that their educational efforts could be skewed towards promoting specific products rather than providing unbiased information. This can lead to an overemphasis on certain treatments at the expense of others, potentially impacting patient care. Ensuring that educational content is evidence-based and free from commercial bias is crucial to maintaining the integrity of medical education.

Navigating the fine line between promotion and education in the pharmaceutical industry requires a careful balance of transparency, regulatory compliance, and ethical considerations. KOLs play a vital role in both areas, and their role must be clarified to maintain the integrity of educational initiatives while recognizing the potential impact of their influence on promotional activities.

Physicians who attend promotional events (dinners, medical symposia, etc.) sponsored by pharmaceutical companies should realize that KOLs are compensated for their presentation and their job is to inform attendees about the benefits and risks of pharmaceutical drugs and devices. They are not permitted to talk off-label, and if asked a question about unapproved uses, they are permitted to give a short and direct answer to the question, but they must return to the on-label, planned presentation. KOLs giving promotional talks are held to the same regulatory standards as pharmaceutical company employees themselves, and they are subject to fines and penalties – and in rare instances, imprisonment – for speaking off-label or disregarding science.

Purely educational content can be funded by pharmaceutical companies but must be developed independently of marketing departments, and peer review and input from a broad range of experts can help maintain the integrity of the information provided. Continuous evaluation of educational programs and feedback from participants can also help ensure that the primary focus remains on education rather than subtle promotion. By prioritizing unbiased, evidence-based information, the industry can better serve healthcare professionals and ultimately improve patient outcomes.

The use of celebrities as key influencers in the pharmaceutical industry can be particularly problematic. Celebrities often lack the medical expertise required to accurately convey the complexities of pharmaceutical products, which can lead to the dissemination of misleading or oversimplified information. This can result in patients making poorly informed decisions based on the perceived authority and popularity of the celebrity rather than on sound medical advice.

The FDA faulted drugmaker AbbVie for misleading claims in a Serena Williams television ad for its migraine medication Ubrelvy. The letter sent by the FDA to AbbVie noted that "[t]he use of a celebrity [tennis] athlete in this TV ad amplifies the misleading representations and suggestions made and increases the potential for audiences to find the misleading promotional communication more believable due to the perceived credibility of the source." The influence of celebrities can also exacerbate issues of accessibility and equity, as high-profile endorsements may drive up demand and prices, making essential medications less affordable for those in need.

I worked in "pharma" for a dozen years. My first job was medical science liaison (MSL). I was hired to provide a company "voice" to KOLs and institutions for products during their life cycle through clinical research and scientific communications – in other words, to influence the influencers. My agenda was based on the business needs of the company.

Many company resources were at my disposal to build strong relationships with KOLs. I was expected to engage in critical peer-to-peer dialogue, provide off-label information when requested, identify "rising stars," support the research process from phases II-IV, and bring clinical feedback to the corporation. The vision of the company was to provide rapid support to KOLs and be the premier field-based medical team of MSLs in the industry.

I left the job after two years. I grew tired of traveling (50-75%). I disliked how the business – in particular, the sales of drugs – prioritized and even determined my activities in the field. And I came to resent the fact that I was calling on KOLs when, in fact, I considered myself a KOL. A narcissistic wound, indeed, because prior to this job, *I* was a well-respected and published academician. MSLs used to call on me! My ego could not bear the reversal of roles.

For my next job (at a different pharmaceutical company), I was hired into traditional R&D. It offered me a better work-life balance and kept me insulated from the marketing department. At the end of the day, however, I realized that whether you are in private practice or working in industry, you can never escape the business realities that dictate the allocation of resources, the necessity for financial viability, and the importance of maintaining operational efficiency.

Due to the extraordinary challenges of psychiatric R&D (high administrative costs, placebo response, etc.), the company stopped doing clinical trials in mental health. Executives determined that psychiatric research had a lower return-on-investment (ROI) compared with other therapeutic areas, such as GI (colitis) and pulmonary (asthma and COPD). They could not justify the financial risks to their shareholders, so they jettisoned psychiatry along with the people doing the research and development. At least I received a severance package.

My third and final job in pharma was special. I joined the company after it had received violations from the FDA for untruthful and misleading advertising. I convinced the hiring manager (and his manager) that the company needed more medical muscle in its internal review of advertising and promotion to ensure scientific accuracy and completeness of information – and I offered to be that muscle! They agreed to let me oversee marketing operations, along with an in-house attorney and a regulatory specialist. I made sure that science and good clinical practices prevailed. The company never received an FDA violation notice during my three years at the helm.

7. Be A Leader Instead of a Micromanager

Empathic, trusting leadership is key to unlocking employees' full potential.

I have worked at many large organizations, and I know how essential it is to be guided by a leader who truly cares for and relates to people rather than one who behaves like a micromanaging boss.

I once worked for a chief medical officer who insisted that everyone on his team email a summary of each day's activities to him. I also worked under a team "leader" who requested the same type of report, only monthly. Another boss insisted on reading and editing clinical summaries I wrote for an insurance company. She persisted in micromanaging my work for two years – needlessly, because all the while she gave me good performance reviews. All three bosses were physicians.

You would think that physicians, with their extensive training and expertise, would be emotionally intelligent, enlightened leaders. However, the reality often diverges from this expectation, as many physicians tend to exhibit micromanagement tendencies. This inclination can stem from various factors inherent in the medical profession.

First, the rigorous training and high stakes associated with patient care instill a deep sense of responsibility in physicians. The desire to ensure that every detail is perfect can lead to micromanagement, as they may feel that delegating tasks could compromise the quality of care. This perfectionist attitude, while beneficial in some respects, can hinder the development of a collaborative and trusting work environment.

Second, the hierarchical structure of the medical field often reinforces micromanagement. Physicians are typically at the top of this hierarchy, which can create a dynamic where they feel compelled to oversee every aspect of patient care. This can lead to a lack of autonomy for other healthcare professionals, such as nurses and physician assistants, who may feel undervalued and underutilized.

Additionally, the intense pressure and workload faced by physicians can exacerbate micromanagement tendencies. The fear of errors and the potential consequences for patient outcomes and attendant malpractice litigation can drive physicians to closely control every aspect of the clinical process. While this approach might mitigate immediate risks, it can stifle innovation and reduce job satisfaction among team members.

Moreover, many physicians receive little to no formal training in leadership and management during their medical education. The focus is primarily on clinical skills and medical knowledge, leaving a gap in essential leadership competencies. Without these skills, physicians may default to micromanagement as a means of maintaining control and ensuring compliance.

Enabling and empowering teams through service, removing barriers (internal and external) and mentoring and coaching trainees through challenges so they mature to face new challenges confidently – that is the kind of leadership that fosters both personal and professional growth.

Still, it fascinates me why people focus on being a micromanaging boss rather than a hands-off leader. The distinctions between them are striking and have significant implications for employee morale and retention. Studies have shown that the leadership qualities of physician supervisors directly impact the well-being and satisfaction of individual physicians working in healthcare organizations (see essay 47).

A micromanaging boss typically holds a position of authority and focuses on maintaining control, enforcing rules, and achieving immediate results. Their approach is often transactional, emphasizing compliance and productivity through directives and monitoring.

In contrast, a leader inspires and motivates their team, fostering a collaborative and inclusive environment. Leaders in health care prioritize long-term goals, such as improving patient outcomes and team development, over short-term gains.

A boss in health care might concentrate on the operational aspects, such as ensuring that staff follow protocols, meet deadlines, and maintain efficiency. This role is crucial for the daily functioning of a medical facility, but it can sometimes result in a rigid work environment where creativity and innovation are throttled. The focus on hierarchy and command can lead to a culture of fear and compliance rather than one of engagement and growth. In contrast, a leader empowers their team, encouraging autonomy and professional development. They cultivate a culture of trust and open communication, where staff feel valued and are motivated to contribute their best.

In the patient care context, the difference between a micromanager and a leader is particularly significant. A boss who micromanages may prioritize metrics such as patient throughput and cost efficiency, potentially overlooking the nuances of patient care and the well-being of the medical staff. This can lead to burnout among healthcare professionals and a decline in the quality of patient care. Conversely, a leader emphasizes the importance of holistic patient care and the mental and emotional health of their team. They understand that high-quality care comes from a motivated, satisfied, and well-supported staff, and they strive to create an environment that nurtures both patients and providers.

Furthermore, in times of crisis, such as during a pandemic, the distinction becomes even more apparent. A micromanager might react with strict rules and pressure, aiming to control the situation through authoritative measures. While this might ensure immediate compliance, it can also lead to heightened stress and reduced morale among healthcare workers. A leader, however, would focus on guiding their team through the crisis with empathy and support, maintaining morale and resilience by fostering a sense of unity and purpose. They communicate clearly and transparently, ensuring that everyone understands the challenges and feels part of the solution.

However, it is important to recognize that the potential for change exists. By fostering leadership development programs that emphasize communication, delegation, and team-building skills, the healthcare industry can help physicians transition from micromanagers to effective leaders. Encouraging a culture of continuous learning and providing opportunities for physicians to engage in leadership training can lead to a more empowered and collaborative healthcare environment.

Ultimately, while the tendency for physicians to micromanage is understandable given the context of their work, addressing this issue through targeted training and cultural shifts can pave the way for more enlightened leadership in healthcare. This shift would not only improve the work environment for all healthcare professionals but also enhance patient care and outcomes.

The table below concludes this discussion with what I believe are some of the key differences between a boss who micromanages and one who leads. I focus on behaviors that, with appropriate coaching, can be modified to instill the best leadership practices and demonstrate that every physician has leadership potential.

Micromanager	**Leader**
Take advantage	Empower
Blame	Fix
Go!	Let's Go!!
Says, "I"	Says, "We"
Intimidate	Rely
Command	Asks
Know how it is done	Show how it is done
Take credit	Give credit

8. The Revolutionary Impact of Artificial Intelligence

AI is transforming the medical landscape in ways that were previously unimaginable.

In a survey of small business owners and employees, both groups said they feel comfortable using artificial intelligence (AI) within their organization to improve customer service, marketing, and sales. A third of business owners said they invested in AI in 2023, and more than half plan to use it in the coming years. Despite the headlines touting AI as a human substitute, most small business owners and employees surveyed viewed the technology as a tool to strengthen and grow their teams rather than replace employees.

The survey, commissioned by Cox Business, included 502 U.S.-based small business owners and 511 U.S.-based small business employees. Most of the investments were in generative AI tools, with the most popular being ChatGPT (other popular tools include Google Gemini, Claude, and Microsoft Bing/Copilot). These tools, which are becoming smarter and faster, use large language models trained to understand information from many different sources to assist workers in daily tasks, enabling them to be more efficient.

For business owners, AI has the potential to sell products, shape and refine business ideas, hone marketing messages, research new topics, and increase productivity by creating and building proposals, writing blogs, designing training material, preparing legal documents, and even writing software code. AI is also seen as a way to support the customer experience, e.g., through online order product/service recommendations; online order placement; website live chatbot; and customer service calls.

There is a corresponding boon in the use of AI in the healthcare industry. The advent of AI in health care has been described as "transformative" and "revolutionary." AI offers numerous benefits and applications that enhance patient care, streamline administrative processes, and advance medical research. In medical imaging and diagnostics, AI algorithms can analyze medical images such as X-rays, CT scans, and MRIs with high accuracy, assisting radiologists in identifying abnormalities like tumors, fractures, or infections. This leads to earlier and more accurate diagnoses. Similarly, AI tools are used in pathology to examine slides, helping pathologists detect diseases such as cancer at a microscopic level more swiftly and accurately.

One of the most impressive uses of AI-assisted imaging involved the use of an AI-powered handheld ultrasonography device operated by novice users. The device estimated gestational age as accurately as credentialed sonographers using ultrasound equipment. Handheld devices are far more affordable than traditional ultrasound equipment, and they could be highly useful in resource-limited settings without expensive ultrasound equipment

Predictive analytics and risk stratification are other areas where AI is making a significant impact (refer to essay 3). AI models can analyze electronic health records (EHRs) to predict which patients are at higher risk of developing certain conditions, such as sepsis, heart disease, or diabetes complications, enabling proactive interventions. Additionally, predictive analytics can identify patients at risk of hospital readmission, allowing healthcare providers to implement targeted strategies to reduce readmission rates.

In the realm of personalized medicine, AI plays a crucial role in genomics by analyzing genetic data to identify mutations and predict responses to treatments, paving the way for approaches tailored to individual genetic profiles. AI can also assist in creating personalized treatment plans by integrating vast amounts of data from clinical trials, medical literature, and patient records to recommend the most effective treatments.

Clinical decision support systems (CDSS) driven by AI provide real-time assistance to clinicians by offering evidence-based recommendations, flagging potential medication errors, and suggesting diagnostic tests or treatments. These systems can also help optimize workflow by prioritizing tasks, managing patient flow, and allocating resources efficiently, thereby improving overall care delivery.

Natural language processing (NLP) is another significant application of AI in healthcare. NLP algorithms can process unstructured data in EHRs, extracting relevant information such as patient histories, symptoms, and treatment outcomes, which can be used for better clinical decision-making and research. AI-powered voice assistants can aid clinicians by transcribing notes, scheduling appointments, and retrieving patient information hands-free, thus reducing administrative burdens.

Robotic process automation (RPA) can automate repetitive administrative tasks such as billing, claims processing, and appointment scheduling, freeing up staff to focus on more complex and patient-centered activities. AI can also optimize inventory management in supply chain management, ensuring that medical supplies are adequately stocked and reducing waste.

In telemedicine and remote monitoring, AI-driven chatbots and virtual assistants can provide patients with medical advice, symptom triage, and appointment scheduling, enhancing access to care. AI-powered wearable devices and sensors can continuously monitor patients' vital signs and health metrics, alerting healthcare providers to any significant changes that may require intervention.

AI is also revolutionizing drug discovery and development. It can expedite the drug discovery process by simulating how different molecules interact, identifying potential drug candidates more quickly and accurately. AI can optimize clinical trial design, patient recruitment, and data analysis, making trials more efficient and cost-effective.

Operational efficiency is greatly enhanced by AI, which can analyze data to predict patient influx, optimizing staff schedules and resource allocation to ensure adequate coverage and reduce wait times. By improving diagnostic accuracy, predicting patient outcomes, and streamlining operations, AI helps reduce healthcare costs.

While AI offers numerous benefits in medicine, there are several downsides that need to be carefully considered. One significant concern is the risk of bias in AI algorithms. If the data used to train these models is not representative of diverse patient populations, the AI may produce biased or inaccurate results, potentially leading to disparities in healthcare outcomes. Additionally, the accuracy and reliability of AI systems are crucial, and errors in AI-driven diagnostics or treatment recommendations could have serious consequences for patient safety.

Another major issue is the challenge of integrating AI into existing healthcare systems. This includes ensuring compatibility with electronic health records (EHRs) and other medical software, as well as providing adequate training for healthcare professionals to effectively use AI tools. Even more fundamental is the role of AI in medical education, given the possibility of plagiarism or simply allowing students to bypass “real” learning.

There are also concerns about data privacy and security, as AI systems often require access to large amounts of sensitive patient information. Ensuring the protection of this data against breaches is paramount. The use of AI in medicine raises additional ethical and regulatory questions, such as determining accountability when AI systems make decisions that adversely affect patient care.

Given that a predominance of AI initiatives is unfolding at a select number of institutions, as we continue to develop and experiment with AI technologies, equitable access to these technologies is crucial to prevent a widening divide in healthcare quality. We must work to ensure that smaller clinics, community hospitals, and underfunded institutions are not left behind. Addressing this challenge is essential to fully realize more inclusive healthcare systems in which AI technologies benefit all patients, regardless of where they are or the resources available to their healthcare providers.

There is no doubt AI in healthcare is revolutionizing the industry by enhancing diagnostic accuracy, personalizing treatments, improving operational efficiency, and expanding access to care. As these technologies continue to evolve, they hold the potential to further transform healthcare delivery, making it more efficient, effective, and patient-centered. However, the integration of AI must be approached with careful consideration of ethical, privacy, and regulatory challenges to ensure that its benefits are realized equitably and safely.

9. Turning Points in Medicine

A segue from Star Trek to D-Day to medical breakthroughs.

I'm a huge fan of Star Trek – the original television series that ran from 1966 to 1969. I've seen each episode many times, and I have all of them on DVD. One of the contenders for "best in franchise" is: "The City on the Edge of Forever," the 28th and penultimate episode of the first season. The script was conceived and mostly written by Harlan Ellison, a prolific and influential author of science fiction and other genres. "City" explores themes of time travel, love, and the moral complexities of altering history.

In this episode, the starship Enterprise encounters temporal disturbances originating from an ancient, sentient time portal known as the Guardian of Forever. During a routine mission, Dr. McCoy accidentally injects himself with an overdose of a powerful drug, causing him to become delusional. In his confused state, he beams down to the planet and jumps through the Guardian, traveling back in time to 1930s Earth. His actions inadvertently alter history, causing the Enterprise to disappear.

Captain Kirk and Mr. Spock follow McCoy through the Guardian to fix the timeline. They arrive in New York City during the Great Depression and discover that McCoy's actions have somehow led to a timeline where the United States did not enter World War II, allowing Nazi Germany to conquer the world. They trace the alteration of history to Edith Keeler (played by Joan Collins), a social worker with visionary ideas for peace. Kirk falls in love with her, but Spock discovers that to restore the original timeline, Edith must die in a traffic accident. If she lives, her pacifist movement delays America's entry into the war, leading to the Nazi victory.

Faced with a moral dilemma, Kirk realizes that he must allow Edith to die to preserve history. In a poignant and heart-wrenching scene, he prevents McCoy from saving her as she steps into the path of an oncoming car. With Edith's death, the timeline is restored, and Kirk, Spock, and McCoy return to the present, where the Enterprise reappears and Kirk snaps, "Let's get the hell out of here."

"The City on the Edge of Forever" represents a crossroads in history within the Star Trek universe by exploring the impact of individual actions on the broader course of events. I watched this episode when the 2024 Olympic games in Paris were taking place. Between swimming and track and field events, NBC featured a short documentary of The Normandy invasion, known as D-Day, a decisive military operation that marked a turning point in the Allied efforts to liberate Europe from Nazi occupation. It was uncanny how the documentary coincided with "City."

I began to think about "turning points" in history – and then medicine – where both the individual and collective actions of doctors and scientists have had life-altering consequences in the course of health care, much like history was altered in Star Trek's "City" and on the beaches of Normandy. Make no mistake, there are key moments in medical history that represent turning points and have significantly changed the trajectory of human health and well-being.

One of the earliest significant milestones was the development of the Hippocratic Corpus in ancient Greece, which laid the foundation for medical ethics and introduced systematic observation and documentation in medical practice. The Renaissance period brought another major turning point with the work of Andreas Vesalius, whose detailed anatomical drawings corrected many of Galen's misconceptions and advanced the understanding of human anatomy.

The advent of the scientific revolution in the 17th century ushered in a new era of medical discoveries. William Harvey's discovery of the circulation of blood in 1628 challenged long-held beliefs and opened the door to modern physiology. In the 19th century, the germ theory of disease, pioneered by Louis Pasteur and Robert Koch, revolutionized the understanding of infection and led to the development of antiseptic techniques by Ignaz Semmelweis (see chapter 14) and Joseph Lister, drastically reducing surgical mortality rates.

The 20th century witnessed groundbreaking advances that further transformed medicine. The discovery of antibiotics, beginning with Alexander Fleming's penicillin in 1928, provided effective treatments for bacterial infections that had previously been fatal. The development of vaccines, such as the polio vaccine by Jonas Salk and Albert Sabin, virtually eradicated diseases that had caused widespread suffering. The introduction of medical imaging technologies, like X-rays, CT scans, and MRI, revolutionized diagnostics, enabling non-invasive visualization of the internal body structures.

Another monumental turning point was the elucidation of the structure of DNA by James Watson and Francis Crick in 1953, which ushered in the era of molecular biology and genetics. This discovery paved the way for the Human Genome Project, completed in 2003, which has had major implications for personalized medicine and the understanding of genetic diseases. The rapid advancement of biotechnology has since led to the development of targeted therapies and gene editing techniques like CRISPR, offering new hope for previously untreatable conditions.

In recent decades, the rise of digital health technologies, including electronic health records, telemedicine, and wearable health devices, has transformed how healthcare is delivered and monitored, enhancing patient engagement and enabling more precise and timely interventions. The COVID-19 pandemic has further accelerated the adoption of these technologies, highlighting their critical role in managing public health crises and ensuring continuity of care.

These turning points, among many others, underscore the dynamic and ever-evolving nature of medicine. Each breakthrough has built upon the knowledge and discoveries of the past, driving progress and improving the quality of life for countless individuals. In essence, while the Normandy invasion and major medical breakthroughs differ in context – one being a military operation and the other a series of scientific advancements – they share common themes of strategic planning, overcoming challenges, decisive impact, lasting legacy, and the embodiment of human endeavor and sacrifice. Both have significantly shaped the course of history and continue to influence the present and future.

As we move forward, continued innovation and interdisciplinary collaboration will be essential in addressing emerging health challenges and advancing the frontiers of medical science. In the inimitable words of Mr. Spock, may we "live long and prosper."

10. The Causes and Consequences of Deception

Deception flourishes where trust and transparency are lacking.

I was deceived countless time in practice, by substance users feigning pain for narcotics and psychiatric patients threatening suicide to gain hospital admission. Deception in medicine is multifaceted, producing signs and symptoms shrouded in ambiguity and mystery. Why do patients deceive physicians and, conversely, why do physicians deceive patients (they do!)? Understanding these dynamics is essential for improving patient outcomes, fostering trust, and maintaining the integrity of the medical profession.

Patient Deception

Patients may deceive their physicians for a variety of reasons, ranging from fear of judgment to financial concerns. One common motivator is the desire to avoid embarrassment or shame. Patients might underreport behaviors such as smoking, alcohol consumption, or drug use due to the stigma associated with these activities. They may fear being judged or receiving a lecture, leading them to provide inaccurate information that can hinder proper diagnosis and treatment.

Another reason for patient deception is the financial burden of healthcare. Patients without adequate insurance coverage might lie about their symptoms or medical history to receive free samples of medications or to avoid additional tests and procedures that they cannot afford. This type of deception can result in suboptimal care and the potential for missed or incorrect diagnoses.

Additionally, some patients may deceive their physicians to obtain certain medications. For instance, individuals with substance use disorders might exaggerate symptoms to receive prescriptions for painkillers or other controlled substances. This not only jeopardizes their health but also contributes to the broader issue of prescription drug abuse.

Malingering, a specific form of deception, describes patients feigning or exaggerating symptoms for secondary gain, such as obtaining disability benefits, avoiding work, or securing drugs (as above). Malingerers can significantly strain healthcare resources, as their deceptive practices often lead to unnecessary tests, treatments, and prolonged clinical evaluations. Identifying malingering is challenging and requires a delicate balance between skepticism and empathy to avoid misjudging genuine cases.

Patients with factitious (not fictitious) disorders, such as Munchausen syndrome, intentionally produce or exaggerate symptoms of illness in themselves to assume the sick role and receive medical attention. Unlike malingerers, their primary motivation is not external gain but rather psychological gratification from being perceived as ill. This form of deception is particularly challenging for healthcare providers because it can lead to extensive and unnecessary medical interventions, which can be harmful to the patient.

The implications of malingering and factitious disorders are significant, often creating ethical challenges to treatments. Both disorders lead to wastage of medical resources and divert attention from patients with legitimate needs. When malingering and factitious disorders are suspected or identified, it can create a sense of betrayal and frustration among medical staff, complicating the therapeutic relationship. Addressing these disorders requires a multidisciplinary approach, including psychiatric evaluation and long-term psychological support.

Emotional Reactions

Physicians' emotional responses to patient deception can be complex and varied. Anger is the main reaction, but it is not the only one. In addition to anger, physicians might feel disappointed, both in the patient and in themselves. They may feel let down by the patient for not being truthful and may also question their own judgment or ability to detect deceptive behavior. However, some physicians, upon understanding the underlying reasons for a patient's deception, may feel empathy and compassion. Recognizing that deception often stems from fear, shame, financial hardship, or psychological issues, they may focus on addressing these root causes rather than reacting with anger.

Concern for patient welfare is another potential reaction and may sometimes override feelings of anger. Many physicians are trained to maintain a level of professional detachment, striving to respond in a calm, measured, and non-judgmental manner. This approach helps maintain the therapeutic relationship and ensures that patient care remains the primary focus.

Reflective practice is another response some physicians may adopt. They may use the experience as an opportunity to consider whether there were any signs they missed or ways to improve communication and trust with patients in the future. Managing emotional responses effectively is crucial, regardless of what physicians may be feeling. Self-awareness is important, as recognizing feelings of anger or frustration can help physicians take a step back and respond more thoughtfully.

Physician Deception

Physicians, too, may engage in deceptive practices, often driven by business pressures or the desire to protect their patients. One significant factor is the pressure to meet administrative and financial targets. In some healthcare systems, physicians are incentivized to see a high volume of patients or to reduce costs. This can lead to practices such as upcoding, where a physician might exaggerate the severity of a patient's condition to receive higher reimbursement from insurance companies. While this may benefit the institution financially, it is illegal and undermines the ethical standards of the profession and can lead to mistrust.

Another form of physician deception is the withholding of information. Physicians might withhold certain details about a diagnosis or prognosis to protect a patient from distress. For example, they might provide a more optimistic outlook on a terminal illness to maintain a patient's morale. While well-intentioned, this paternalistic approach can prevent patients from making fully informed decisions about their treatment and end-of-life care.

Furthermore, physicians may sometimes deceive patients by overstating the benefits of certain treatments or downplaying potential risks. This can occur due to a physician's belief in the efficacy of a treatment or due to external pressures from pharmaceutical companies. Such deception can lead to patients undergoing unnecessary or harmful procedures, eroding trust in the medical profession.

And for reasons that are only known to physicians, themselves, they may deceive the public at large. For example, Emily Marantz, MD, an ob/gyn practicing in New Jersey, reportedly posed as a man named "Ethan" and maintained intimate online chats with women on an internet dating site. Sociologist Anna Akbari, PhD, wrote about her involvement with "Ethan" in her memoir, *There Is No Ethan*. None of the women roped into Marantz' deception ever received a satisfactory explanation as to why she would do this, although clearly her behavior would question Marantz' reliability as a physician. Her intimate online deception of women is especially concerning, given that Marantz is a gynecologist.

Even more alarming, sometimes physicians have resorted to severe, lethal forms of deception, as discussed in essay 39.

Implications for the Medical Profession

Deception, whether by patients or physicians, has significant ramifications for the medical profession. For patients, deceptive practices can lead to misdiagnoses, inappropriate treatments, and ultimately poorer health outcomes. For physicians, engaging in or being subjected to deception can compromise professional integrity and contribute to burnout and moral distress.

Building a healthcare environment rooted in trust and transparency is the solution. Physicians must foster open communication, encouraging patients to share accurate information without fear of judgment. This can be achieved through empathetic listening, patient education, and creating a non-judgmental atmosphere. Ongoing education and training in areas like patient communication, behavioral health, and ethics can equip physicians with tools to handle deception more effectively.

Similarly, healthcare systems must address the systemic pressures that incentivize deceptive practices among physicians, promoting ethical standards and patient-centered care. By understanding the motivations behind deceptive behaviors in general and issues that contribute to and maintain deception, the healthcare community can work towards a more honest, transparent, and effective system of care.

11. Diversity Action Plans for Clinical Trials

A critical evaluation of the FDA's guidance reveals opportunities and challenges for sponsors.

The FDA is intent on improving the enrollment of participants – also known as "subjects" – from underrepresented populations in clinical studies involving drugs and devices. The FDA's initiative is not unlike the attempts of institutions of higher learning to increase student diversity through diversity, equity, and inclusion (DEI) programs. The FDA has issued guidance for sponsors – mainly the pharmaceutical industry – entitled "Diversity Action Plans to Improve Enrollment of Participants from Underrepresented Populations in Clinical Studies."

Clinical studies assess the safety and efficacy of drugs and devices designed for preventing, treating, or diagnosing various conditions and diseases. In the U.S., certain populations are often underrepresented in biomedical research despite bearing a disproportionate burden of specific conditions. This underrepresentation stems from multiple factors, such as assumptions about the feasibility of enrolling a representative population and the potential impact on study timelines, as well as the absence of a proactive strategy to ensure the enrollment and retention of a study population that mirrors the intended use population.

Toward Inclusivity

The FDA's draft guidance emphasizes the creation of Diversity Action Plans (DAPs) aimed at ensuring the enrollment and retention of a clinically relevant study population that accurately represents various age groups, sexes, and racial and ethnic demographics. Nevertheless, the FDA acknowledges the wider issues of health disparities and unequal access to healthcare and clinical studies, which can be influenced by factors such as geographic location, gender identity, sexual orientation, socioeconomic status, physical and mental disabilities, pregnancy and lactation status, and comorbidities. The FDA encourages sponsors of clinical studies to consider these additional factors when developing their DAPs.

It should be noted that FDA guidance documents – and there are many of them on a range of topics – describe the Agency's current thinking on a topic and are to be viewed only as recommendations, unless specific regulatory or statutory requirements are cited.

The FDA's guidance on DAPs marks a significant advancement towards enhancing inclusivity and representation in clinical trials. The guidance provides a well-structured and detailed framework for sponsors to develop and implement DAPs. By specifying elements such as enrollment goals disaggregated by race, ethnicity, sex, and age, the FDA ensures that sponsors consider a wide range of demographic factors. This comprehensive approach is essential for addressing disparities in clinical research and ensuring that study results are applicable to diverse populations.

The guidance's suggestions for practical measures to reduce participant burden – such as transportation assistance, dependent care, and flexible hours for study visits – are particularly valuable. These recommendations can significantly enhance participation from underrepresented groups who may face logistical challenges in attending study visits.

Additionally, the encouragement of decentralized clinical trials (DCTs) is a forward-thinking approach. DCTs permit participants to complete parts or all of the clinical study at home, essentially bringing the clinical trial personnel and equipment to the participant rather than requiring participants to undergo evaluation at study sites. DCTs can increase accessibility for participants who are geographically distant from study sites, thereby enhancing the diversity of the study population. This aligns with the broader trend towards using technology to make clinical research more inclusive.

How to Improve the FDA's Guidance

The guidance requires sponsors to monitor enrollment goals and provide updates in annual reports, which ensures ongoing accountability. This continuous oversight can help identify and address barriers to meeting diversity goals in real-time, potentially leading to more successful outcomes.

However, implementing the guidance may pose challenges, especially for smaller sponsors or those with limited resources. The additional administrative burden of developing, submitting, and regularly updating DAPs could be significant, and sponsors may need extra support and resources to comply effectively. Although the guidance is robust, some areas could benefit from greater clarity. For instance, the criteria for waivers from DAP requirements are outlined, but the process for obtaining such waivers might be further detailed to prevent ambiguity. Including more specific examples or case studies could also help sponsors understand how to meet enrollment goals effectively.

Implementing the recommended measures, such as providing transportation assistance and dependent care, could increase the costs of conducting clinical trials. While these measures are essential for improving diversity, they may also impact the overall budget and feasibility of clinical studies, particularly for smaller companies. Moreover, the guidance emphasizes the importance of monitoring enrollment goals but is less clear on the enforcement mechanisms if sponsors fail to meet these goals (probably because FDA guidance documents are not binding). More stringent enforcement policies or incentives for compliance could strengthen the effectiveness of the DAP requirements.

The Impact of More Diverse Study Populations

By promoting the inclusion of diverse populations in clinical trials, the guidance can enhance the generalizability of study results. This is crucial for ensuring that medical products are safe and effective for all segments of the population, not just those historically overrepresented in clinical research. Increased transparency and efforts to include underrepresented populations can improve public trust in the clinical research process, which is particularly important given the historical mistrust among certain demographic groups towards medical research (think: Tuskegee Syphilis Study).

The emphasis on DCTs and reducing participant burden could drive innovation in clinical trial design and execution. Sponsors may develop new strategies and technologies to meet these requirements, potentially leading to more efficient and inclusive clinical research practices.

In conclusion, the FDA's guidance on DAP represents a significant and necessary step forward in promoting inclusivity in clinical research. While comprehensive and well-intentioned, its implementation may pose challenges, particularly for smaller sponsors. Enhancements in clarity, support for implementation, and enforcement mechanisms could further strengthen its impact. Overall, the guidance has the potential to significantly improve the representation of diverse populations in clinical trials, thereby enhancing the generalizability and applicability of medical research outcomes.

12. Mistrust Towards Medical Research

The roots of distrust among ethnic minorities date back centuries.

In the previous essay, I alluded to the historical mistrust among certain demographic groups towards medical research. It is a deeply rooted issue, stemming from a legacy of exploitation, unethical practices, and systemic discrimination. This mistrust has significant implications for public health, as it can lead to underrepresentation of ethnic minorities in clinical trials and healthcare disparities. Understanding the origins and perpetuation of this mistrust is crucial for developing strategies to rebuild trust and ensure equitable healthcare outcomes.

The Tuskegee Syphilis Study

One of the most notorious examples of unethical medical research is the Tuskegee Syphilis Study, conducted by the U.S. Public Health Service between 1932 and 1972. In this study, 600 African American men in Tuskegee, Alabama, were recruited under the guise of receiving free healthcare. Of these, 399 had syphilis, and 201 did not. The men were not informed of their diagnosis and were denied effective treatment, even after penicillin became widely available as a cure in the 1940s. The study aimed to observe the natural progression of untreated syphilis, resulting in severe health consequences and death for many participants.

The Tuskegee Syphilis Study is a tragic example of medical exploitation and deception, significantly contributing to the mistrust African Americans have towards medical institutions. The revelation of the study in 1972 led to public outrage, legal settlements, and eventually, the establishment of stricter ethical standards in medical research, including the requirement of informed consent.

In essence, the Tuskegee Experiment violated the principles of the Nuremberg Code, a set of ethical guidelines developed in response to the unconscionable medical experiments conducted by Nazi doctors during World War II. In effect, the Nuremberg Code stipulates that:

- Research participants must give informed consent
- Research must be conducted in a way that minimizes harm
- Research must be based on scientific validity

The long-lasting impact of this study continues to influence the perception of medical research within the African American community. This was particularly evident during the COVID-19 pandemic and the related reluctance in communities of color to get vaccinated.

The Exploitation of Henrietta Lacks

Another significant case is the story of Henrietta Lacks, an African American woman whose cancer cells were taken without her knowledge or consent in 1951. These cells, known as HeLa cells, became one of the most important tools in medical research, contributing to numerous scientific breakthroughs, including the development of the polio vaccine, cancer treatments, and in vitro fertilization techniques. Despite the immense scientific value of HeLa cells, Lacks and her family were neither informed nor compensated, raising serious ethical questions about consent and the exploitation of African American patients.

The story of Henrietta Lacks underscores the broader issues of consent and the exploitation of marginalized groups in medical research. It highlights the need for transparency, respect, and compensation, and continues to fuel mistrust among African Americans towards the medical research community.

The Guatemala Syphilis Experiments

Another egregious example is the Guatemala Syphilis Experiments, conducted by the U.S. government between 1946 and 1948. In these experiments, American public health doctors deliberately infected Guatemalan prisoners, soldiers, and psychiatric patients with syphilis and other sexually transmitted infections without their informed consent. The purpose was to test the effectiveness of penicillin. The subjects were not informed of the nature of the experiments or given adequate treatment, resulting in severe health consequences for many.

The Guatemala Syphilis Experiments reflect the broader pattern of unethical medical practices conducted on vulnerable populations, often outside the United States. These experiments contribute to the mistrust of medical research not only within the Guatemalan community but also among other Latin American populations who may view medical research as exploitative and harmful.

Medical Experimentation on Native Americans

Native American populations have also been subjected to unethical medical research practices. In the mid-20th century, the U.S. government conducted involuntary sterilizations on Native American women, often without their knowledge or consent. Additionally, Native American children were used in nutritional experiments in residential schools, where they were deliberately malnourished to study the effects of dietary supplements.

These practices have left a lasting legacy of mistrust towards medical and governmental institutions among Native American communities. The historical trauma associated with these unethical practices continues to impact their willingness to participate in medical research and trust healthcare providers.

Other Instances of Medical Exploitation

The historical record is replete with other instances of medical exploitation and unethical research practices targeting marginalized groups. For example, during World War II, Japanese scientists conducted horrifying experiments on Chinese prisoners of war, including vivisections and biological warfare tests. In the United States, the Cold War era saw numerous unethical experiments, such as the exposure of military personnel to radiation without their informed consent.

Implications for Contemporary Medical Research

The historical mistrust towards medical research among certain demographic groups has significant implications for contemporary health care. As discussed in the prior essay, it can lead to underrepresentation of certain groups in clinical trials, which in turn effects the generalizability of research findings and the development of treatments that are effective across diverse populations. This underrepresentation can perpetuate health disparities and hinder efforts to achieve health equity.

To address this mistrust, it is essential to implement measures that ensure transparency, informed consent, and respect for participants' autonomy. Building trust requires acknowledging past wrongs, providing reparations where appropriate, and actively involving marginalized communities in the research process. Community engagement, culturally competent care, and the inclusion of diverse researchers and healthcare providers are also critical components of rebuilding trust. Only by acknowledging past transgressions and committing to equitable and respectful treatment can the medical research community hope to rebuild trust and achieve more inclusive and representative healthcare outcomes.

13. Unethical Legacies in Medical History

Reexamining legacy and revoking reverence help restore medical integrity.

In 2021, U.S Congress ordered the Defense Department to look into renaming military bases, ships, and anything else that was named in honor of Confederate figures. The Naming Commission recommended changing the names of nine Army bases and Navy ships.

Even more recently, my college dormitory at Boston University, Myles Standish Hall, was renamed "610 Beacon Street" – its physical address. Standish provided military muscle for the Pilgrims and notoriously ambushed and slaughtered Native Americans at a supposedly peaceful summit.

In recent years, there has been a growing movement to reevaluate and often rename medical programs, buildings, statues, and other honors that bear the names of physicians and professionals whose past actions or beliefs are now considered unethical or harmful. This mirrors the broader societal shift towards acknowledging and rectifying practices considered racist, sexist, discriminatory, and dehumanizing.

But is this trend justified? It can be difficult to draw the line between condemning unethical behavior and recognizing valuable contributions when looking back in time. Additionally, such actions could lead to a slippery slope where historical figures are judged solely by contemporary standards, potentially leading to the erasure of important aspects of history. Thus, some institutions have instead chosen to keep the names of certain individuals in question but add plaques or exhibits that provide a fuller context, acknowledging both their achievements and ethical failings.

Let's look at a few instances where a naming overhaul felt warranted to those in charge.

One prominent example is the legacy of J. Marion Sims, MD, often referred to as the "Father of Modern Gynecology." Sims developed pioneering surgical techniques in the 19th century, but his methods included performing experimental surgeries on enslaved African American women without anesthesia and without their consent. Such practices, viewed through the lens of contemporary ethical standards, are deeply troubling. As a result, a statue of Sims was removed from Central Park in New York City in 2018.

Similarly, the name of Thomas Parran Jr., MD, a former Surgeon General, has come under scrutiny. Parran played a significant role in public health advancements, but he was the intellectual inspiration of the infamous Tuskegee Syphilis Study that I discussed in the previous essay. Due to his involvement, the University of Pittsburgh renamed Parran Hall, which previously housed the Graduate School of Public Health. The American Sexually Transmitted Diseases Association (ASTDA) renamed the Thomas Parran Award as "The ASTDA Distinguished Career Award."

Several other esteemed physicians have had their names removed from an award or edifice. Joseph DeJarnette, MD, had his name taken off a Virginia mental health facility in 2001 after it was discovered he had championed Nazi eugenics policies and supported increased sterilization efforts in the U.S.

More recently, the "Father of Space Medicine" fell to earth when allegations of the involvement of Hubertus Strughold, MD, in Nazi concentration camp medical experiments earned greater credibility. The controversy caused the Space Medicine Association to end the annual presentation of an award given in Strughold's honor. His name was dropped from a plaque on a building façade, and his portrait was removed from a gallery at Ohio State University.

The legacy of Hans Asperger, MD, an Austrian pediatrician after whom Asperger syndrome was named, has also been reexamined. Recent historical research has uncovered Asperger's complicity with Nazi eugenics policies, including his involvement in the euthanasia of disabled children. This has led to a reconsideration of the use of his name in medical diagnoses. The Diagnostic and Statistical Manual of Mental Disorders (DSM-5-TR) eliminated Asperger's disorder, which is now subsumed under the general heading of autism spectrum disorder.

Several other Nazi and Nazi-sympathizing physicians have been discredited and had their names removed from the medical lexicon and disorders that once bore their names:

- Julius Hallervorden, Hallervorden-Spatz disease, neurodegeneration;
- Hans Eppinger, Cauchois-Eppinger-Frugoni syndrome, portal vein thrombosis;
- Hans-Joachim Scherer, van Bogaert-Scherer-Epstein disease;
- Hans Seitelberger, Seitelberger disease, infantile neuroaxonal dystrophy;
- Hans Scherer, van Bogaert-Scherer-Epstein syndrome, cerebrotendinous xanthomatosis;
- Eduard Pernkopf, seven-volume anatomical atlas;
- Friedrich Wegener, Wegener syndrome;
- Hans Reiter, Reiter syndrome, reactive arthritis

These efforts are part of a broader movement within the medical community and society at large to critically assess the legacies of historical figures whose contributions to science and medicine are overshadowed by their unethical actions or beliefs. Renaming diseases, programs, buildings, and statues is seen not only as a way to rectify past wrongs, but also as a means to ensure that the names honored in public spaces reflect values of equity, justice, and respect for all individuals.

Promoting moral standards is the key outcome of this process. Reexamining legacy helps identify practices and individuals whose actions may not meet today's ethical standards, encouraging a shift towards honoring those who have made positive contributions without ethical compromises. By revoking reverence for those whose actions are deemed unethical by modern standards, the medical community reinforces the importance of integrity and ethical behavior within the profession.

Fostering diversity, equity, and inclusion is also achieved through this critical reassessment. Reexamining legacy allows for the recognition of previously overlooked contributions from diverse and marginalized groups, promoting a more inclusive and accurate historical narrative. Addressing and correcting past biases through revoking reverence helps create a more equitable environment that respects the contributions of all individuals, regardless of their background.

The educational impact of this process is significant. Reexamining legacy – and providing context for various acts of renaming – provides an opportunity to educate current and future medical professionals about the complexities of medical history, including both its achievements and ethical failings. Revoking reverence works to incorporate ethics in medical school curricula.

Restoring public trust is another vital benefit of reexamining legacy and revoking reverence. Transparent reassessment of historical figures and practices builds public confidence in the medical profession's commitment to ethical standards. By taking a stand against unethical behavior, the medical community can demonstrate that the profession holds itself accountable to the highest standards. Professional – or personal – silence in the face of social injustice is wrong.

While prominent figures may have made significant contributions to the medical field, their actions and beliefs must be scrutinized in light of their impacts on vulnerable populations. By reexamining legacy, revoking reverence, and instituting corrective measures, the medical community can uphold its commitments to equity and ethical inquiry.

14. "Character Assassination" in Medicine

The consequences of unjustly targeting clinicians affect patients and institutions too.

Character assassination refers to the deliberate and sustained effort to damage someone's reputation or credibility through false or misleading accusations, innuendo, or manipulation of information. This can be done through various means, including spreading rumors, exaggerating faults, or attributing malicious motives to a person's actions. The goal is often to undermine the individual's standing, influence, or career.

In politics, attacking the character of an opponent has become a familiar refrain. But character assassination also occurs in medicine and other professions. In medicine, it can manifest in several ways. Professional rivalries in highly competitive environments, such as academia or hospital administration, might lead colleagues or competitors to engage in character assassination to discredit one another and gain an advantage. This can include spreading rumors about someone's competence, ethics, or personal behavior.

Medical professionals who expose unethical practices, patient safety issues, or financial fraud may become targets of character assassination as a form of retaliation. Attempts to discredit the whistleblower can include questioning their motives, competence, or mental stability.

Physicians involved in medical errors or malpractice cases can face character assassination as part of legal strategies. Opponents may attempt to portray the physician as negligent or incompetent, regardless of the actual circumstances. In some medical settings, character assassination can be a tactic used in workplace bullying.

This can involve spreading false information about a colleague to undermine their professional standing, isolate them socially, or force them out of their position.

High-profile cases or media coverage can sometimes lead to character assassination of medical professionals. Sensationalist reporting or biased narratives can unfairly tarnish a physician's reputation based on incomplete or inaccurate information. For example, animosity towards Anthony Fauci, MD, reigned supreme as the coronavirus pandemic wore on, and although it did not play a significant role in his decision to leave his position at the White House, Republicans vowed to investigate him. Fauci said he would consider testifying before Congress, but he would not submit to "character assassination."

Admiral Rachel L. Levine, MD, a pediatrician and longtime leader in public health, was sworn in as assistant secretary for health at HHS in March 2021. She made history as the first openly transgender federal official to be confirmed by the U.S. Senate – barely confirmed by a vote of 52-48. During the confirmation, Levine faced hostile and, at times, transphobic questioning from senators. Other politicians have made hateful remarks about her on social media while stoking fear and lies about gender-affirming care for youth. "People fear what they don't understand," Levine remarked, vowing to protect the health rights of Americans and trans individuals.

Bennet Omalu, MD, MBA, MPH, is a Nigerian-American forensic pathologist who discovered chronic traumatic encephalopathy (CTE) in American football players. His findings, which linked repeated head trauma to severe brain damage, were initially met with intense opposition from the National Football League (NFL) and some members of the medical community. Efforts to discredit his research and reputation included questioning his credentials and motives. Despite these attacks, Omalu's work eventually gained acceptance and led to significant changes in how concussions are managed in sports.

Ignaz Semmelweis, MD, a Hungarian physician in the 19th century, discovered that handwashing with chlorinated lime solutions drastically reduced the incidence of puerperal fever among obstetric patients. Despite his findings, Semmelweis faced severe backlash from the medical community. His colleagues ridiculed and ostracized him, largely because his ideas conflicted with the established medical beliefs of the time. His reputation was so tarnished that he eventually lost his position and was committed to an asylum, where he was beaten by guards and died 2 weeks later from a gangrenous wound that may have been caused by the beating.

Frances Oldham Kelsey, MD, PhD, was a pharmacologist and physician who worked for the FDA as a medical reviewer. In the early 1960s, she resisted pressure from pharmaceutical companies to approve thalidomide (Thalomid), which was already available in dozens of countries around the world. The drug, used for morning sickness in pregnant women, was later found to cause severe birth defects. Kelsey's steadfast refusal to accept inadequate safety data and bow to industry pressure (in the form of drug executives complaining bitterly to her superiors) ultimately saved countless lives and led to stronger drug regulation policies.

There are many other healthcare professionals whose characters were assassinated simply for insisting on scientifically reliable evidence and telling the truth.

The consequences of character assassination in medicine can be severe, affecting not only the targeted individual's career and mental health but also patient care and institutional integrity. It can lead to loss of job opportunities, professional isolation, legal battles, and emotional distress. Fauci quickly encountered problems in his role, realizing that former President Donald Trump "was saying things that were just not true" about COVID-19 treatments. Fauci and his family faced credible death threats for handling the response to the pandemic.

Preventing and addressing character assassination in medicine requires a robust support system, including strong professional ethics; cultivating an atmosphere of integrity and respect within medical institutions; implementing clear policies and procedures to address and resolve conflicts, bullying, and retaliation; providing protection and support for those who raise legitimate concerns; ensuring fair and transparent investigations; and offering mental health resources for those affected.

By fostering a supportive and ethical work environment, medical institutions can help mitigate the risks and impacts of character assassination.

15. The Impact of the Legal Profession on the Practice of Medicine

Ongoing dialogue and collaboration between the legal and medical professions is essential for addressing complex healthcare issues, ensuring patient safety, and fostering a more integrated approach to public health and health delivery.

Long ago, a mentor told me to write my patients' progress notes like they might be read one day aloud in a deposition. Her advice is no less true today than it was decades ago. It serves as an important reminder for all healthcare professionals that accurate, detailed documentation isn't just a task – it's a safeguard. Progress notes today could be scrutinized in the future, potentially impacting legal outcomes, patient care, and professional reputations. Always chart with precision and clarity, knowing that the future might hold those words to a higher standard.

My mentor's advice was aimed squarely at the intersection of medicine and the law, which has shaped the landscape of healthcare in both beneficial and challenging ways. Historically, the relationship between law and medicine has evolved through various key events, creating a complex dynamic that continues to evolve today.

In the early 20th century, the establishment of medical licensing laws marked a significant turning point. These laws, designed to standardize medical education and practice, were instrumental in ensuring that only qualified individuals could practice medicine. This regulatory framework not only helped to protect patients from unqualified practitioners but also elevated the overall standards of medical care. Additionally, this period saw the development of malpractice laws, which aimed to provide recourse for patients harmed by negligent medical care. These laws, while initially rudimentary, laid the groundwork for more comprehensive legal protections for patients in the future.

The mid-20th century brought about significant advancements in medical technology and treatment, necessitating more sophisticated legal oversight. The rise of medical malpractice litigation in the 1960s and 1970s, driven by high-profile cases and increased public awareness, underscored the need for legal mechanisms to address medical errors and patient safety. This period saw the introduction of informed consent laws, which required physicians to fully disclose the risks and benefits of treatments to their patients. This legal requirement not only empowered patients to make more informed decisions about their healthcare but also fostered greater transparency and trust in the physician-patient relationship.

However, the increasing prevalence of malpractice litigation also had negative repercussions. The fear of legal action led to the practice of defensive medicine, where physicians, concerned about potential lawsuits, ordered unnecessary tests and procedures to protect themselves from liability. This practice not only increased healthcare costs but also sometimes subjected patients to unnecessary risks and interventions. The legal profession's influence thus introduced a tension between safeguarding patient rights and the unintended consequences of over-cautious medical practice.

Taken to the extreme in mental health, the safeguarding of patients' rights often backfired. Patients defended by vigorous counsel were allowed to be discharged from hospitals unable to properly care for themselves as long as they did not present a clear and present danger to others. Dark humor circulated that discharging homeless patients in the wintertime allowed them to freeze to death, but at least their civil liberties were intact.

One critical area where the law and medicine began to intersect was evident is in the doctrine of the "corporate practice of medicine." This legal doctrine restricts corporations or non-physicians from practicing medicine or employing physicians to provide medical services. The intent behind this doctrine is to ensure that medical decisions are made in the best interest of patients, free from commercial pressures and conflicts of interest that could arise if non-medical entities were involved in the delivery of healthcare. However, this doctrine has been challenged and modified over time, leading to variations in its application across different states. In some regions, exceptions have been carved out, allowing certain corporate entities, such as hospitals and health maintenance organizations (HMOs), to employ physicians directly, provided that medical decisions remain the purview of licensed medical professionals.

In tandem with the corporate practice of medicine, "safe harbor laws" play a pivotal role in shaping the legal landscape of healthcare. These laws provide protections for healthcare providers against certain legal actions, provided they comply with specified standards or regulations. For instance, safe harbor provisions may shield physicians from liability under anti-kickback statutes if they adhere to strict guidelines designed to prevent financial incentives from influencing medical decisions. These laws are designed to foster an environment where healthcare providers can focus on patient care without the constant threat of legal repercussions, provided they operate within the boundaries of established legal and ethical standards. By offering these protections, safe harbor laws aim to balance the need for regulatory oversight with the necessity of allowing healthcare professionals to practice medicine without undue interference.

The National Practitioner Data Bank (NPDB) has significantly influenced the practice of medicine, specifically in relation to the legal profession's impact. Established in 1986, the NPDB serves as a repository of information regarding medical malpractice payments, adverse licensure actions, and other negative actions taken against healthcare practitioners. This database aims to enhance the quality of healthcare by restricting the ability of incompetent practitioners to move from state to state without disclosure of their previous performance.

In the late 20th and early 21st centuries, the legal profession continued to shape medical practice through the enactment of further healthcare laws and regulations. The Health Insurance Portability and Accountability Act (HIPAA) of 1996 is a prime example, establishing stringent standards for patient privacy and the protection of medical information. While these regulations have been crucial in safeguarding patient confidentiality, they have also introduced administrative burdens on healthcare providers, requiring significant investments in compliance and data management systems.

More recently, the Affordable Care Act (ACA) of 2010 represented a landmark legal intervention in the healthcare system, aiming to expand access to healthcare and reduce costs. The ACA's provisions, such as the establishment of health insurance exchanges and the expansion of Medicaid, have had widespread impacts on the practice of medicine. These changes have increased the number of insured patients, thereby increasing demand for medical services. However, the complexities of navigating the new legal and regulatory environment have also posed challenges for healthcare providers, requiring adaptations in practice management and patient care delivery.

Throughout this timeline, the legal profession has played a dual role in the practice of medicine. On the positive side, legal interventions have been pivotal in promoting patient safety, ensuring high standards of medical care, and protecting patient rights. Laws and regulations have driven improvements in medical practice, fostering greater accountability and transparency. On the negative side, the fear of litigation and the administrative burdens of compliance have sometimes hindered the efficiency and effectiveness of medical practice. The practice of defensive medicine and the complexities of regulatory compliance have introduced challenges that healthcare providers must continually navigate.

The legal profession's impact on the practice of medicine highlights the intricate balance between legal oversight and medical autonomy (see essay 20). While laws and regulations have been essential in safeguarding patient welfare and enhancing the quality of care, they have also introduced challenges that necessitate ongoing adaptation and resilience within the medical community. This evolving relationship underscores the need for continued dialogue and collaboration between the legal and medical professions to ensure that the healthcare system serves the best interests of patients and providers alike.

Efforts to foster continued communication between the legal and medical professions are multifaceted, encompassing educational initiatives, policy reforms, interdisciplinary committees, and integrated practice models. Here are some of the key steps being taken:

1. **Interdisciplinary Education and Training:** Medical and law schools increasingly recognize the importance of interdisciplinary education. Joint degree programs, such as MD/JD programs, and specialized courses that cover medical ethics, healthcare law, and policy are becoming more prevalent. These programs aim to equip future professionals with a comprehensive understanding of both fields, fostering mutual respect and collaboration.
2. **Continuing Professional Development:** Ongoing professional development opportunities for practicing physicians and lawyers include seminars, workshops, and conferences focused on the intersection of law and medicine. These events often feature case studies, panel discussions, and collaborative problem-solving sessions that address current legal and medical issues.

3. **Policy and Advocacy:** Professional organizations, such as the American Medical Association (AMA) and the American Bar Association (ABA), actively engage in policy advocacy. They work together to influence legislation and regulatory reforms that impact healthcare delivery. These organizations also create task forces and committees to address specific issues, such as medical malpractice reform and patient privacy regulations.
4. **Integrated Practice Models:** Integrated practice models, such as Accountable Care Organizations (ACOs) and Patient-Centered Medical Homes (PCMHs), promote collaboration between healthcare providers and legal professionals. These models encourage a team-based approach to patient care, where legal experts are involved in addressing complex issues related to compliance, risk management, and patient rights.
5. **Mediation and Alternative Dispute Resolution:** To address the adversarial nature of malpractice litigation, there is a growing emphasis on mediation and alternative dispute resolution (ADR) methods. These approaches aim to resolve conflicts between patients and healthcare providers more amicably and efficiently, reducing the stress and costs associated with traditional litigation.
6. **Tort Reform:** ADR is a major component of tort reform, which encompasses a variety of strategies aimed at improving the medical malpractice system, for example, caps on damages, limits on attorney fees, and pretrial screening panels or medical review boards to evaluate the merits of malpractice claims before they proceed to court. The goal of tort reform is to reduce the frequency and severity of litigation, lower malpractice insurance premiums, and ultimately reduce the burden of litigation.
7. **Health Law Research and Scholarship:** Academic research centers and think tanks dedicated to health law and policy play a crucial role in analyzing the impact of legal issues on healthcare. These institutions conduct studies, publish

reports, and provide evidence-based recommendations to inform policy decisions and improve the legal framework governing medical practice.

8. **Collaborative Technology Platforms:** Advancements in technology have facilitated better communication and collaboration between legal and medical professionals. Electronic health records (EHRs) and secure communication platforms enable real-time sharing of information, ensuring that legal considerations are integrated into clinical decision-making processes.
9. **Public Health Initiatives:** Joint public health initiatives, such as those addressing the opioid crisis, mental health, and infectious diseases, require close collaboration between legal and medical professionals. These initiatives often involve coordinated efforts to implement and enforce public health laws, provide education and resources to communities, and ensure access to necessary medical and legal services.

These steps reflect a concerted effort to bridge the gap between the legal and medical professions, fostering a more cohesive and effective healthcare system. By continuing to build on these initiatives, both fields can work together to address emerging challenges and ensure that patient care remains at the forefront of their collaborative efforts.

16. Strange Bedfellows: The Complex Relationship Between Law and Medicine

Interdisciplinary collaboration, shared education, and a focus on common goals make the relationship work.

The term "strange bedfellows" originates from a line in Shakespeare's play *The Tempest*, written in 1611. In Act 2, Scene 2, the character Trinculo says, "Misery acquaints a man with strange bedfellows." This phrase has come to describe unlikely alliances or partnerships between individuals or groups with differing backgrounds, interests, or viewpoints.

The fields of law and medicine are often considered "strange bedfellows" due to their complex and sometimes uneasy interactions, as touched upon in the previous essay. These professions have fundamentally different goals and perspectives. Medicine primarily focuses on patient care, healing, and improving health outcomes, driven by the principles of beneficence (doing good) and non-maleficence (doing no harm). In contrast, the legal profession emphasizes justice, fairness, and the protection of legal rights, operating under principles of accountability, liability, and the rule of law. This divergence in focus can create tensions, particularly when the goals of healing and justice seem to conflict.

The nature of each profession also contributes to this perception. Law often operates within an adversarial framework, especially in litigation, where opposing parties contest issues in a competitive environment. Medicine, on the other hand, generally functions within a collaborative framework, with healthcare providers working as a team to deliver the best possible care to patients. This fundamental difference in approach can lead to misunderstandings and friction between the two fields.

In psychiatry, this tension can be particularly pronounced. Psychiatrists aim to provide compassionate and patient-centered care, often working collaboratively with other healthcare professionals to develop comprehensive treatment plans for individuals with mental health disorders. However, when psychiatric patients become involved in legal matters – such as competency hearings, involuntary commitments, or criminal cases – the adversarial nature of the legal system often clashes with the therapeutic goals of psychiatry.

The absurdity of strange bedfellows can sometimes manifest in humorous ways, as illustrated by this vignette. I was required to extend the involuntary commitment of one of my patients who had not improved after several days in the hospital. The hearing took place in a makeshift courtroom within the hospital. My patient's counsel was prepared to argue against the extension. Suddenly, the patient erupted, refusing to participate in the hearing. He began shouting, "There's no American flag. It's not a real courtroom." Recognizing the severity of the patient's psychosis, despite his statement being true, the hearing official granted an additional 21 days of commitment without a formal proceeding.

Risk management is another area where the law and medicine diverge. Medical practice involves managing clinical risks and uncertainties, often requiring rapid decision-making based on incomplete information. Legal practice, conversely, involves managing legal risks and liabilities, necessitating meticulous documentation, evidence collection, and adherence to procedural rules. The impact of malpractice litigation further complicates the relationship. Medical professionals may feel that the threat of litigation creates a defensive practice environment, leading to over-testing, over-treatment, and increased healthcare costs. Legal professionals might argue that malpractice litigation is necessary to hold healthcare providers accountable and ensure patient safety (refer to the previous essay).

Communication styles also differ significantly between the two fields. Medical communication often relies on clinical jargon, shorthand, and a focus on patient symptoms, diagnosis, and treatment plans. Legal communication emphasizes precise language, detailed documentation, and a focus on statutes, regulations, and case law. These differences can create barriers to effective collaboration and mutual understanding. Physicians are fond of saying that medical school teaches the language of medicine. Lawyers say the same about law school – it teaches the language of law.

Despite these differences, law and medicine are not entirely incompatible. Both professions ultimately aim to serve the public interest. Medicine seeks to improve health and save lives, while law seeks to protect rights and ensure justice. These shared goals can create common ground for collaboration. Increasingly, healthcare delivery and legal frameworks are becoming intertwined, necessitating interdisciplinary collaboration. Issues like patient consent, confidentiality, and end-of-life decisions require input from both medical and legal professionals.

Both fields operate under strict ethical guidelines and professional standards. Medical ethics (e.g., the Hippocratic Oath) and legal ethics (e.g., the ABA Model Rules of Professional Conduct) emphasize principles of integrity, responsibility, and respect for individuals. This shared commitment to ethics can foster mutual respect and understanding. Lawyers and doctors can work together to advocate for patient rights and improve healthcare policies. Legal professionals can help navigate complex healthcare regulations, while medical professionals provide the necessary clinical expertise.

Joint educational programs and interdisciplinary training can also bridge the gap between the two fields. Programs that educate medical professionals about legal issues and vice versa can promote mutual understanding and respect. The specialties of psychiatry and pathology offer training and sub-specialization in the field of forensics, certified by the American Board of Medical Specialties. Furthermore, collaborative efforts in policy-making and healthcare reform demonstrate that law and medicine can work together to address systemic issues. Public health initiatives, for instance, often require coordinated legal and medical responses.

Finally, there are physicians who become lawyers, and vice versa. The transition from physician to lawyer is more common than the reverse. Physicians who become lawyers often do so to gain expertise in areas such as malpractice litigation, healthcare policy, and regulatory compliance, in order to advocate more effectively within the healthcare system. I've known several MD/JDs who've used their dual education as a pathway to chief executive positions within health care.

While law and medicine may seem like "strange bedfellows" due to their differing approaches, goals, and methodologies, they are not entirely incompatible. The intersection of these two fields is essential for addressing many complex issues in modern society. Through interdisciplinary collaboration, shared education, and a focus on common goals, law and medicine can work together to enhance patient care, uphold justice, and improve public health outcomes.

17. The Anti-Psychiatry Movement

Opposition to psychiatry should be balanced with the greater good, considering the essential role of psychiatrists in diagnosing, treating and preventing mental disorders.

A college student wrote: "Part of the goal of psychiatry (and the psychiatric colonial assault) functions to replace an embodied and intergenerational value system, beliefs, and invisible web of culturally attuned knowledge and traditions that support a sense of self and community and identity." Essentially, the student was critiquing psychiatry from the perspective that it can act as a tool of cultural domination, potentially erasing valuable cultural knowledge and traditions.

The student's background from Hawaii provides a significant context to understand and validate their perspective. Hawaii has a unique cultural heritage and history, including the impact of colonialism and the resulting tension between traditional Hawaiian practices and Western influences. This context lends weight to the student's critique of psychiatry from the viewpoint of cultural preservation and autonomy. It also relates to themes from the larger anti-psychiatry movement that emerged in the 1960s and 1970s, questioning the fundamental assumptions, practices, and power structures of mainstream psychiatry.

The anti-psychiatry movement is characterized by its diverse and often radical nature, condemning the legitimacy of psychiatric diagnoses, the ethics of psychiatric treatments, and the power dynamics inherent in the doctor-patient relationship, which may be magnified in the psychiatric field. It draws from a variety of intellectual traditions, including existentialism, sociology, and the field of medical anthropology, influenced by broader social movements advocating for civil rights and personal liberation.

One of the central figures in the anti-psychiatry movement was Thomas Szasz, MD (1920-2012), whose seminal work *The Myth of Mental Illness* argued that mental illnesses are not real diseases but rather constructs used by society to control and stigmatize individuals who deviate from normative behaviors. Szasz contended that psychiatric labels are often employed to enforce social conformity and that the coercive practices of psychiatry, such as involuntary hospitalization and forced medication, violate individual autonomy and human rights. His critique extended to the very language of psychiatry, which he believed pathologized normal human experiences and emotions.

Another influential voice was R.D. Laing (1927-1989), a Scottish psychiatrist whose work focused on the lived experiences (see essay 33) of individuals diagnosed with schizophrenia. Laing challenged the traditional view that schizophrenia was a biological disorder, instead proposing that it was a meaningful response to an untenable social and familial environment. His book *The Divided Self* emphasized understanding patients' subjective experiences and argued for a more empathetic and humanistic approach to mental health care. Laing's ideas resonated with the countercultural movements of the 1960s (see essay 22), which championed personal freedom and questioned established authorities.

Michel Foucault (1926-1984), the French philosopher and social theorist, also contributed significantly to the anti-psychiatry discourse with his historical analysis of the development of psychiatric institutions. In *Madness and Civilization*, Foucault traced the history of how societies have defined and treated madness, revealing how psychiatric practices have often been used as tools of social control. He argued that the rise of the asylum represented a shift in the management of deviance, from punishment to medicalization, and highlighted the power imbalances between those labeled as mentally ill and the authorities who confine and treat them.

The Church of Scientology is known for its strong anti-psychiatry stance. Since its inception, the Church has been vocally critical of psychiatry, viewing it as a harmful and pseudoscientific practice. This opposition is rooted in the teachings of Scientology's founder, L. Ron Hubbard (1911-1986), who denounced psychiatric treatments and institutions as abusive and detrimental to individuals' mental and spiritual well-being. Hubbard's views are outlined in his book *Dianetics: The Modern Science of Mental Health*, published in 1950. This book introduces the core concepts of Dianetics, which later evolved into the broader framework of Scientology.

The anti-psychiatry movement was not merely an academic exercise; it had practical implications and led to the establishment of alternative mental health practices. For example, Scientology's anti-psychiatry position is institutionalized through organizations like the Citizens Commission on Human Rights (CCHR), which the Church established in 1969. The CCHR campaigns against psychiatric practices, particularly the use of psychiatric medications and procedures such as electroconvulsive therapy (ECT). It argues that these treatments are often coercive and harmful, promoting instead Scientology's own, controversial methods for addressing mental health issues.

The therapeutic communities pioneered by figures like R.D. Laing and South African psychiatrist David Cooper (1931-1986), who coined the term "anti-psychiatry," sought to create environments where patients could live more freely and engage in more egalitarian relationships with caregivers. These communities emphasized mutual support, non-coercion, and the importance of social context in mental health recovery. The movement also influenced the development of patient advocacy groups and the broader mental health consumer movement, which sought to give voice to those with lived experience of mental health issues and to promote reforms in mental health care systems.

Critics of the anti-psychiatry movement argue that it sometimes downplays the suffering associated with severe mental illnesses and fails to acknowledge the benefits that psychiatric treatments, including medications, can provide for many individuals. They also point out that while the movement has effectively highlighted the need for greater empathy and respect in mental health care, it has not always offered practical alternatives to biomedical approaches, nor has it recognized irrefutable scientific findings that show that fundamentally, serious mental illnesses such as schizophrenia and bipolar disorder, stem from disorders of the brain.

There have been significant efforts within the field of psychiatry to address and rectify previous criticism. Professional organizations such as the American Psychiatric Association (APA) and the Royal College of Psychiatrists have played pivotal roles in advocating for the scientific and clinical value of psychiatry. These organizations work to enhance public understanding of mental health issues through educational campaigns that emphasize the effectiveness of psychiatric treatments, the importance of mental health care, and the medical training of psychiatrists. Indeed, psychiatry residents' "match" numbers have been increasing yearly since 2011 (see essay 49), and in 2023 psychiatry was one of just 10 specialties with increases of more than 10% over the past five years.

Research initiatives funded by government agencies and private institutions aim to advance the field by developing new therapies and improving existing ones, thereby demonstrating the tangible benefits of psychiatric care. Additionally, mental health professionals engage in public discourse through media appearances, publications, and community outreach to dispel myths and misinformation propagated by anti-psychiatry advocates.

Collaborative efforts with patient advocacy groups such as the National Alliance on Mental Illness (NAMI) also help to amplify the voices of those who have benefited from psychiatric care, providing personal testimonies that counteract negative perceptions. These combined efforts strive to foster a more informed and supportive environment for mental health treatment, ultimately promoting the greater good by ensuring access to effective and compassionate psychiatric care.

18. Post-Hospitalization Disparities in Health Care

Equity-informed policies and health system strategies are needed to reduce gaps in care.

We often hear that "a rising tide lifts all ships," but when it comes to health care, that tide isn't lifting everyone equally. As highlighted in a 2024 article from the *Annals of Internal Medicine*, the care patients receive after leaving the hospital is just as crucial as the therapy they receive within it. Unfortunately, disparities in treatment – prior to hospitalization, during hospitalization, and post-hospitalization – appear be worsening, leaving vulnerable populations even further behind.

The study showed significant variation and disparities in follow-up care for Medicare beneficiaries treated in the hospital for acute myocardial infarction and heart failure. The largest disparities were between Black and White patients, but Asian and Hispanic patients were impacted as well. The article underscores a critical aspect of healthcare that often goes overlooked: the continuum of care that extends beyond the hospital walls.

The research highlights the importance of comprehensive patient management, recognizing that the quality of care patients receive after discharge is integral to their overall health outcomes. This notion is particularly pertinent in light of the growing disparities in healthcare, which seem to be exacerbating across the entire spectrum of medical treatment.

Prior to hospitalization, individuals from marginalized communities often face barriers such as limited access to primary care, inadequate health education, and financial constraints. These barriers contribute to the progression of untreated conditions, leading to more severe health issues by the time hospitalization becomes necessary. During hospitalization, disparities can manifest through differential treatment, biased clinical decision-making, and varying levels of access to advanced medical technologies. These inequities do not cease at discharge; they continue to affect the quality of post-hospitalization care.

Post-hospitalization, patients from underserved communities frequently encounter obstacles that hinder their recovery. These include limited access to follow-up care, inadequate health literacy, and social determinants of health such as unstable housing and food insecurity. Furthermore, the healthcare system's fragmentation often means that critical information is lost in transition, and continuity of care is disrupted. For instance, a patient discharged with specific instructions for managing a chronic condition may not have the means to afford necessary medications or medical equipment, or may lack transportation to attend follow-up appointments. These gaps in care disproportionately affect vulnerable populations, perpetuating a cycle of poor health outcomes and readmissions.

Addressing these disparities requires a multifaceted approach that involves healthcare providers, policymakers, and community organizations. Healthcare providers must adopt a more holistic view of patient care, one that extends beyond the hospital stay. This includes developing comprehensive discharge plans that consider the patient's social and economic context, ensuring clear communication of care instructions, and facilitating connections to community resources. Additionally, leveraging technology such as telemedicine can help bridge gaps in access, providing remote monitoring and consultation for patients who might otherwise lack follow-up care.

Policymakers play a crucial role in reducing healthcare disparities by enacting policies that promote equitable access to care. This includes expanding insurance coverage, increasing funding for community health programs, and incentivizing healthcare providers to serve in underserved areas. Moreover, efforts to address social determinants of health through broader social policies – such as affordable housing, education, and employment opportunities – are essential in creating an environment where all individuals can achieve optimal health.

Community organizations also have a significant part to play in supporting post-hospitalization care. These organizations can provide critical services such as patient education, transportation assistance, and home health visits. By fostering partnerships between hospitals and community groups, we can create a more integrated care network that supports patients throughout their recovery journey.

Effective recovery doesn't end at discharge. However, the essential elements to bridge the gap between hospital and home are not accessible to everyone. As a result, disparities in treatment are occurring across the healthcare continuum, and they highlight a pressing need for systemic change. By addressing the social determinants of health, improving access to care, and ensuring continuity of care, we can build a more equitable healthcare system that supports all patients, particularly those from disadvantaged populations. Let's work together to ensure that every patient has the support they need to fully recover, no matter where they start – and end.

19. Political Incursions in the Doctor-Patient Relationship

How to give identity politics a proper voice in the doctor-patient relationship.

I don't recall politics being as contentious and prominent as it was during the 2024 Presidential election. I never anticipated hospitals would rally patients to register to vote, or that a healthcare provider would write in a patient's chart, "We again discussed … the importance of voting and the safety, security, and effectiveness of voting by mail." However, considering the sharp political divides across the U.S., I suppose it was to be expected.

It seems there is already too much medical information to cover during a 10 to 15-minute primary care visit to include discussions about politics. Nevertheless, politics – identity politics in particular – has found a medical voice, underscoring the importance of striving for a healthcare system that is inclusive, equitable, and responsive to the realities of all patients.

"Identity politics" refers to political positions and perspectives that are based on the interests and viewpoints of social groups with which people identify. These groups can be defined by various characteristics such as race, gender, sexuality, religion, or other markers of identity. The core idea is that individuals from these groups advocate for policies and social changes that address their specific needs and experiences, often in response to historical and systemic inequities.

In recent years, identity politics has increasingly infiltrated the medical field. There is a presumption that doctors should be as concerned with politics as they are with medicine. A study of 44 countries, including the U.S., found that people who were registered to vote tended to report better subjective health than those who did not vote or participate in civic activities, according to findings published in the *Journal of Preventive Medicine & Public Health.*

Close associations between politics and medicine can be seen in several ways. First, medical education and training programs are placing greater emphasis on cultural competence and sensitivity to diversity. This includes understanding how social determinants of health, such as race and socioeconomic status, impact patient outcomes. Curricula are increasingly addressing topics like implicit bias, health disparities, and the importance of providing equitable care to all patients. (At the same time, however, some universities have eliminated diversity, equity and inclusion [DEI] offices or made sweeping cutbacks to their programs.)

Second, there is a growing recognition within the healthcare community of the need to address health disparities and inequities. Professional organizations and advocacy groups are pushing for policies that aim to reduce these disparities, such as expanding access to healthcare for marginalized groups and addressing social determinants of health.

Third, physicians are becoming more aware of the importance of considering a patient's identity in their care. This can mean being sensitive to how a patient's background might affect their health and their interactions with the healthcare system. It also involves creating an inclusive and welcoming environment for all patients, regardless of their identity, and refraining from posts on social media that could be viewed otherwise.

Fourth, there is an increasing focus on collecting and analyzing data related to health outcomes across different identity groups. This helps in identifying and addressing health disparities. Research funding and priorities are also shifting to ensure that studies include diverse populations and consider the impact of identity on health. Public health initiatives are becoming more tailored to address the specific needs of different identity groups. This targeted approach aims to improve health outcomes by considering the unique challenges and barriers faced by these groups.

While the incorporation of identity politics into the medical field aims to create a more equitable healthcare system, it also brings challenges. These include navigating potential conflicts between different identity groups, balancing individual patient needs with broader social goals, and ensuring that efforts to address disparities do not inadvertently stigmatize or marginalize certain populations.

The question of whether doctors should discuss politics with their patients invites strong opinions on both the "left" and "right" sides. Liberals and conservatives essentially make the same arguments, i.e., physicians must protect patients from radical, divisive ideology, while arguing from extreme and opposite viewpoints.

Professional boundaries are a key consideration in this issue. The primary role of a physician is to provide medical care and support to their patients. Discussions should generally center around the patient's health, treatment options, and well-being. Introducing political discussions could potentially alienate or distress patients, which might damage the trust and rapport that are essential for an effective doctor-patient relationship.

Ethical considerations also play a significant role. Physicians should avoid causing harm, adhering to the principle of non-maleficence. Political discussions can be polarizing and may inadvertently cause emotional or psychological distress to patients. Additionally, as I discuss in the following essay, respecting a patient's autonomy involves acknowledging their right to their own beliefs and values, which includes political views.

The situational context may sometimes necessitate political discussions, particularly when political issues directly impact patient health, such as policies on healthcare access, reproductive rights, and gender identity. In such cases, it might be appropriate to discuss these topics in a way that is informative and relevant to the patient's care. If a patient initiates a political discussion and it is relevant to their concerns or care, a physician could engage, but should do so carefully, ensuring the discussion remains respectful and professional.

Practically, physicians might find it best to maintain a neutral stance if political topics arise, focusing on how policies may affect health and well-being rather than expressing personal political opinions. If a political discussion starts to become contentious, it may be helpful to gently steer the conversation back to the patient's health and care.

While there may be instances where discussing political matters is relevant and necessary, it should be approached with caution, always prioritizing the patient's health, comfort, and the integrity of the doctor-patient relationship. In my experience, however, most patients will welcome the conversation and appreciate that their doctors are interested in aspects of their life beyond a diagnosis.

20. The Erosion of Patient Autonomy

Balancing autonomy and treatment have become as much a moral as a medical issue.

The erosion of patient autonomy is a growing concern in contemporary health care, manifesting in several critical clinical areas. One prominent example is reproductive health, where access to abortion has been increasingly restricted, thereby limiting women's ability to make autonomous decisions about their bodies and reproductive futures (see essay 37). These constraints not only infringe upon personal freedoms but also complicate the physician-patient relationship, as doctors may find themselves unable to offer comprehensive care due to legal limitations.

Another significant area is end-of-life care. Euthanasia and physician-assisted suicide remain unavailable in most states, leaving terminally ill patients with limited options to end their suffering on their own terms. This lack of autonomy can lead to prolonged suffering and a diminished quality of life, as patients are forced to endure conditions that they would otherwise choose to escape through medically assisted means.

Sports medicine, particularly concerning repeated concussions and suicidality in professional football players, also highlights the tension between patient autonomy and medical paternalism. While the intention behind banning repeatedly concussed players is to protect their long-term health, it can be seen as an infringement on their autonomy. These athletes may wish to continue their careers despite the risks, yet are often prevented from doing so by medical regulations aimed at preserving their future well-being, decreasing the possibility of chronic traumatic encephalopathy (CTE). (One in three former living National Football League players believe they have CTE, according to a Harvard study.)

These examples underscore a broader trend of diminishing patient autonomy in healthcare, which has far-reaching implications for patients, families, the public, and the medical community. Additionally, there are numerous other instances making headlines recently, such as:

1. **Involuntary Commitment and Treatment**: Patients with severe mental illnesses, such as schizophrenia or bipolar disorder, may sometimes be involuntarily committed or subjected to treatment without their consent. This raises significant ethical concerns about autonomy, especially when patients disagree with the diagnosis and treatment, or refuse to accept treatment. The balance between ensuring patient safety, the safety of the public, and respecting patient autonomy is delicate and fraught with moral complexities.
2. **Opioid Prescribing Restrictions**: In response to the opioid crisis, many regulations have been implemented to limit opioid prescriptions. While these measures aim to curb addiction and misuse, they can inadvertently restrict access to necessary pain relief for patients with various pain syndromes. This creates an ethical dilemma where the autonomy of patients to choose their pain management strategy is compromised, potentially leading to untreated pain and decreased quality of life.
3. **The Rights of Parents vs. Adolescents**: The question of who has the right to make healthcare decisions – the adolescent or the parents – can lead to ethical conflicts. For instance, in cases where an adolescent desires gender reassignment therapy, but the parents refuse all possible interventions, the healthcare team must navigate the complex interplay between respecting the emerging autonomy of the adolescent and the legal rights of the parents, as well comply with state laws that may prevent gender-assisted therapy.
4. **Mandatory Vaccinations**: Public health policies mandating vaccinations for preventable diseases raise ethical questions

> about individual autonomy versus community health. While these policies aim to protect public health, they can infringe on personal autonomy and the right to make individual healthcare decisions. This is particularly contentious in cases where individuals have strong personal or religious beliefs against vaccinations.

The encroachment upon patient autonomy can be attributed to a variety of factors, including legislative actions, medical guidelines, and institutional policies that prioritize safety and public health over individual choice. While the intention behind these measures is often to protect patients from harm, they can inadvertently strip individuals of their right to make informed, independent decisions about their own health and well-being.

The principle of autonomy is a cornerstone of medical ethics, emphasizing the importance of respecting patients' rights to make decisions about their own bodies and medical treatments. When autonomy is compromised, it challenges the very foundation of trust and mutual respect that is essential for effective patient-physician relationships.

Furthermore, the balance between protecting patients and respecting their right to self-determination becomes increasingly precarious. On one hand, healthcare providers have a duty to prevent harm and promote the best possible outcomes for their patients. On the other hand, patients have the right to make choices that align with their personal values, beliefs, and preferences, even if those choices involve certain risks and run counter to the advice of clinicians.

This tension is particularly evident in the clinical areas discussed above, where the stakes are high and the consequences of restricting autonomy are potentially detrimental. For instance, limiting access to abortion not only affects women's health but also their socioeconomic status and overall life trajectory. Similarly, denying terminally ill patients the option of euthanasia can lead to unnecessary suffering and a loss of dignity in their final days. In sports medicine, prohibiting athletes from continuing their careers due to health risks may protect them from future harm but also denies them the opportunity to pursue their passions and livelihoods.

The erosion of patient autonomy has significant implications not only for the patients themselves but also for their family members. When patients are unable to make independent decisions about their healthcare, the burden often shifts to family members who may find themselves in challenging and emotionally charged positions. For instance, in the context of reproductive health, when women are denied access to abortion, it can place immense strain on families, both emotionally and financially. Family members may have to support a loved one through an unplanned pregnancy or navigate the complexities of raising a child in difficult circumstances, which can alter family dynamics and impact overall well-being.

In end-of-life care, the lack of access to euthanasia or physician-assisted suicide can also deeply affect family members. They may be forced to witness prolonged suffering and a diminished quality of life in their loved one, leading to emotional distress and feelings of helplessness. Family members often play a crucial role in the caregiving process, and when patients are unable to exercise their autonomy in making end-of-life decisions, it can result in prolonged caregiving responsibilities that can be physically, emotionally, and financially draining. Moreover, families may face difficult ethical dilemmas and disagreements about the best course of action, which can strain relationships and permanently break psychological bonds.

In the realm of sports medicine, particularly concerning repeatedly concussed athletes, family members may also bear the weight of these decisions. While medical professionals may restrict an athlete's participation to safeguard their health, families must cope with the emotional fallout. Athletes who are forced to retire due to health concerns may experience a loss of identity and purpose, which can lead to mental health issues such as depression and anxiety. Family members often become the primary support system, managing the emotional and psychological repercussions while also grappling with their own fears and concerns for their loved one's future.

The trend is now unmistakable. Patients' rights to self-determination are being encroached upon by multiple stakeholders. Individuals are no longer in control of their own health. Practitioners may not honor patients' decisions as broader societal issues eclipse their wishes. But look at it on the bright side. There has never been a more opportunistic time for healthcare providers, policymakers, and politicians as a whole to engage in ongoing dialogue and reflection to ensure that the rights and well-being of patients are upheld while also safeguarding public health and safety.

21. The Growing Preference for Texting in Healthcare Encounters

Supplanting telephone conversations with text messages has benefits – and challenges –especially in the elderly.

Surely, if there were to be a sequel to *E.T. The Extra-Terrestrial*, the famous line “E.T. phone home” would be updated to “E.T. text home.”

There is no doubt that texting has largely replaced telephone conversations as the dominant mode of social communication today. This shift can be attributed to several factors. Texting offers greater convenience, allowing people to communicate at their own pace without the immediate pressure of a live conversation. It also facilitates asynchronous communication, enabling individuals to respond when it suits them, which is particularly useful in busy or noisy environments. Additionally, texting supports multitasking, making it easier to integrate into daily routines.

The preference for texting is especially strong among younger generations, such as millennials and Gen Z, who often favor it over phone calls. This trend has influenced broader communication habits. Moreover, texting is viewed as a more informal and less intrusive way to connect, making it the preferred method for quick updates, questions, or casual conversations. While phone calls remain important for urgent, personal, or detailed discussions, texting has become the primary mode of communication in many social settings.

It is no surprise, therefore, that healthcare systems are putting significant effort and resources into designing patient portals to help patients become more engaged in their care, and the most frequently utilized feature of portals is secure text messaging. Texting is the most interactive and collaborative feature of patient portals and most likely to facilitate increased patient engagement with their providers and their care.

Many in the health professions attest to secure messaging due to its convenient and efficient way to exchange information. Patients can easily inquire about their health information, ask questions, request prescription refills, and discuss test results without the need for phone calls or in-person visits. This can lead to more timely interventions and better overall management of chronic conditions. Additionally, secure messaging can improve the documentation and continuity of care, as all communications are recorded and can be referenced as needed.

A family medicine physician wrote, "Adopting secure messaging not only has helped [our practice] provide more satisfying, efficient, and effective patient care with no more hassle, but it also has helped us meet the National Committee for Quality Assurance's requirements for patient-centered medical home certification, which has helped us obtain higher reimbursements from certain payers." The physician had initially assumed that patients weren't ready for secure messaging or that, if they were, it would overburden staff. "We couldn't have been more wrong," she concluded.

However, despite obvious advantages of secure messaging, there are significant pitfalls. One major concern is the potential for breaches of patient confidentiality and data security. Even though these systems are designed to be secure, they are not immune to hacking and cyber-attacks. Unauthorized access to sensitive health information can have serious consequences, including identity theft and loss of patient trust.

Furthermore, the convenience of secure messaging can sometimes lead to an overwhelming volume of messages for healthcare providers, contributing to burnout and reducing the time available for direct patient care. Miscommunication and misunderstanding can also occur more easily in written messages compared to face-to-face interactions, potentially leading to errors in diagnosis or treatment.

Messages may go unchecked when a healthcare provider is on vacation, and staff may fail to notify patients and establish a coverage system when providers are away. Patients may message providers expecting a quick reply despite usual disclaimers within portal systems that emergency concerns should not be left in a message, as well as language asking patients to allow 24 to 48 hours for a reply.

The loss of personal touch that telephone conversations can provide is probably the biggest drawback to messaging. Voice communication allows for immediate clarification of questions and concerns, and the nuances of tone and inflection can convey empathy and understanding in a way that written messages often cannot. This is particularly important in psychiatry, where the therapeutic relationship and the ability to convey empathy are crucial components of patient care. Moreover, some complex or sensitive issues might be more appropriately handled through a direct conversation rather than through written messages.

Additionally, not all patients are equally comfortable or proficient with digital communication tools, or have the means to utilize them, which can create barriers to access and understanding. As mentioned above, while younger, tech-savvy patients may prefer electronic messaging, older adults or those with limited access to technology might find it challenging. This digital divide can exacerbate disparities in healthcare access and quality.

Yet, despite barriers, studies show that older patients seem to want to use electronic means of communicating with their physicians. Although enthusiasm to use email, in particular, among older adults tends to decrease with increasing age, it still remains relatively high overall. Promoting the use of computerized portals and secure messaging to older adults requires certain adaptations. These should include ease of use, direct provider contact, and reassurances that access and interpersonal relationships will not be sacrificed to electronics.

It is also essential to address the mental health concerns of older adults because anxiety and depression may decrease the acceptance of text messaging. Between 2019 and 2023, there was a rise in mental health diagnoses – primarily anxiety and depressive disorders – among older adults, with a 57.4% increase in those aged 65 and older. Given this context, it is important to consider how the increased prevalence of mental health issues in older adults makes the adoption of new technologies challenging.

The unfamiliarity with digital communication tools, compounded by the potential stress or confusion associated with learning and using these systems, could also act as a barrier. However, with the right support and adaptations, these barriers can be mitigated. Providing comprehensive training and user-friendly guides can help older adults become more comfortable with portal systems. Additionally, offering reassurance and ongoing assistance from healthcare providers and support staff can alleviate anxiety related to using new technology.

It is important to emphasize the potential benefits of using portal systems for mental health support. For instance, secure messaging can provide a convenient and less intimidating way for older adults to reach out to their healthcare providers, especially when discussing sensitive mental health issues. While many patients still value in-person visits for complex or serious health concerns, where a physical examination and direct conversation are crucial, they sometimes prefer texting to discuss topics they find uncomfortable to address in person.

Ultimately, while the rise in mental health diagnoses among older adults presents challenges, it also highlights the critical need for accessible and supportive communication channels. By addressing these barriers thoughtfully and providing robust support systems, healthcare providers can help older adults navigate portal systems effectively, ensuring they receive both the physical and mental health care they need.

22. The Long Strange Trip of Psychedelic Drugs

Despite decades of research, there is no FDA-approved psychedelic agent.

In the mid-1960s, the Grateful Dead were the house band for Ken Kesey's Acid Tests, parties in which people were "tripping out" on LSD, parties that helped bring psychedelics into the counterculture. Psychedelic drugs have been the focus of extensive clinical research since then, and their potential therapeutic benefits have seen renewed interest in recent years. It's been a long strange trip for certain because, despite extensive research, there are currently no FDA-approved psychedelic medications on the market.

The initial wave of psychedelic research in the 1960s was not only closely tied to counterculture movements, it was endorsed and funded by the CIA, which was looking for a mind control drug. However, experimentation with psychedelics, whether sanctioned or not, led to political and social backlash and the classification of many psychedelics as Schedule I substances under the Controlled Substances Act in 1970. This classification severely restricted research and development, and lingering concerns have plagued the process ever since. The *BMJ* placed an expression of concern on a meta-analysis about a methodological error that likely overestimated the benefits of psilocybin for treating symptoms of depression.

The most recent blow was dealt by an FDA advisory committee meeting in June 2024. The Psychopharmacologic Drugs Advisory Committee voted 9-2 that the available data failed to show MDMA, commonly known as ecstasy, was effective in treating patients with PTSD. And by a vote of 10-1, it was deemed that its risks outweighed the benefits, even with a proposed risk evaluation and mitigation strategy (REMS). The FDA was not bound to accept the recommendations of the Committee; nevertheless, two months later, it declined to approve the treatment without another study and other stipulations.

The rigorous process of FDA approval involves multiple phases of clinical trials to demonstrate safety and efficacy, and psychedelics present unique challenges in designing and conducting these trials due to their complex effects on the brain. One significant challenge is clinical trial design, particularly with regard to functional unblinding, a situation in clinical trials where participants and/or researchers can infer which treatment a participant is receiving, despite efforts to maintain blinding.

Psychedelics typically produce intense and unmistakable psychoactive effects, such as altered perception, mood, and cognition. These effects are usually quite different from those of a placebo, making it relatively easy for both participants and researchers to guess whether a participant has received the active drug or a placebo. This awareness can introduce bias, as participants' expectations and researchers' observations may be influenced, potentially skewing the trial's results.

Addressing functional unblinding in psychedelic research often requires innovative trial designs. Some strategies include using active placebos (substances that produce mild psychoactive effects but are not expected to have therapeutic benefits) or incorporating more rigorous and objective outcome measures that are less susceptible to bias. These approaches aim to preserve the blinding and ensure that the results of the trial are reliable and valid. Moreover, the FDA's own regulatory code outlines several other study design options that could be used.

Another hurdle in psychedelic research is the difficulty in finding the "ideal agent." Different psychedelics have varying effects, durations, and safety profiles. Identifying a compound that offers the most therapeutic benefit with the least risk is a complex and ongoing process. The leading contenders today in clinical trials are MDMA, psilocybin, and LSD. Apart from their powerful psychological effects, some may have significant effects on blood pressure, heart rate, and rhythm.

Additionally, the therapeutic use of psychedelics often requires a combination of the drug with psychotherapy. This integrated approach, sometimes referred to as psychedelic-assisted therapy, necessitates trained therapists and specialized settings, further complicating the clinical trial process and eventual implementation in standard clinical practice.

It is generally accepted that most clinical trials involving the use of psychedelics should be conducted by academics and in conservative, safe environments. However, this has not allayed concerns about misconduct during the trials – underreporting of serious adverse events and, in one incident, alleged sexual misconduct by an unlicensed therapist with a patient – prompting the scientific journal *Psychopharmacology* to retract three papers for "protocol violations amounting to unethical conduct" by the researchers.

Ethical concerns do indeed play a significant role in psychedelic research. The hallucinogenic effects of psychedelics can lead to challenging experiences, and there is a moral responsibility to ensure that participants are not harmed. This includes thorough screening, informed consent, and providing adequate support during and after the experience, which is why a REMS program would most certainly be a requirement of any FDA-approved agent. Researchers are also hopeful that the FDA will clarify how psychotherapy should be utilized in future psychedelic trials.

Historically, limited funding for psychedelic research due to stigma and regulatory barriers has been an issue, though this is beginning to change as more private and public entities recognize the potential benefits of these substances. Recent studies have shown promising results in treating conditions such as depression, PTSD, and substance use disorders. Organizations like MAPS (Multidisciplinary Association for Psychedelic Studies) and academic institutions are conducting rigorous research to build a strong evidence base.

Growing interest from patients and the public in alternative treatments for mental health conditions is driving demand for further research and potential approval of psychedelic therapies. Considering only PTSD, there are 13 million Americans who live with the disorder, and there have been no new drug treatments this century (the FDA approved sertraline and paroxetine for PTSD in 1999). While there are no FDA-approved psychedelic medications currently available, the landscape is rapidly evolving, and ongoing research, increasing funding, and shifting societal attitudes may pave the way for future approvals and broader acceptance of psychedelics in clinical practice.

23. Peer-to-Peer Review – Part 1

Physicians should insist on specialty-specific reviews if they are second-guessed by insurance companies.

A significant number of physicians frequently find themselves engaged in "peer-to-peer" reviews with insurance companies. These reviews are a burdensome step to secure approval for medications or procedures deemed medically necessary for their patients. However, there is a widespread concern among doctors regarding the qualifications of the health plan-appointed peers conducting these reviews. Many practicing physicians report that these appointed peers often lack the appropriate qualifications to make informed decisions about the specific medical needs of their patients. This discrepancy can lead to delays in treatment, harm to patients, and additional administrative burdens on physicians.

A peer-to-peer review typically involves a telephone discussion between a practicing physician and an insurance company physician (or representative) to determine whether a medical service or prescription medication is medically necessary, not experimental, and a benefit covered by the health plan. It's bad enough that the health plan physician has no first-hand knowledge of the patient; it's worse yet to discover that they may not be a true "peer."

In a 2023 survey by the American Medical Association (AMA), just 15% of 1000 physicians said that the health plan-appointed peer "often" or "always" have the appropriate qualifications. More than one-third of physicians said that payer peers "rarely" or "never" have the expertise required to make a medical necessity determination. That means, for example, that a breast oncologist could end up talking to a "peer" who is an ob-gyn and unfamiliar with the nuances of treating breast cancer. Sometimes, the peer isn't even a physician.

Bruce A. Scott, MD, is president of the AMA (until June 2025) and an otolaryngologist in private practice in Louisville, Kentucky. He is all too familiar with the frustration of not being able to speak to a physician who understands his specialty. Writing in an AMA Leadership Viewpoints column, Dr. Scott observed: "I sit down with a patient, listen to their history, do a thorough exam, review imaging studies and then together we decide on a treatment plan. But then I have to get approval from an insurance company representative who has never seen my patient and who typically isn't even a physician. Never mind an otolaryngologist who could best understand the prescribed course of treatment; it's rare the person on the other line can even pronounce otolaryngology."

The concept of a "peer" in the context of peer-to-peer reviews ideally means a physician with similar training, expertise, and experience as the treating physician. For a health plan-appointed physician to be considered a true peer, they must possess specific qualifications that align closely with the specialty and subspecialty of the treating doctor. For instance, if the treating physician is a psychiatrist (like me), the insurance company physician should also be a board-certified psychiatrist with substantial clinical experience in the field of psychiatry – not a psychologist or social worker. This ensures they have a comprehensive understanding of the nuances and complexities involved in treating patients with psychiatric and medical disorders.

Moreover, if I subspecialized in child and adolescent psychiatry, the health plan should provide a psychiatrist with additional board certification in child and adolescent psychiatry. Children are not "little adults." Specialized understanding is crucial for making informed decisions about their treatment plans, medication management, and therapeutic interventions tailored to the developmental stages and specific mental health issues of this younger population.

Having recent and relevant clinical practice experience is also important. A physician actively engaged in patient care is more likely to be up-to-date with the latest medical advancements, treatment protocols, and emerging best practices. This current clinical involvement equips them with a practical perspective on patient management, which is essential for making informed decisions during the review process. This is no different than many jurisdictions which require that physicians who serve as expert witnesses be actively practicing or have practiced within a recent time frame.

Additionally, the reviewing physician should typically manage the medical condition or disease in question or provide the healthcare service under peer-review consideration. This ensures they have direct experience and expertise in handling similar cases, which is critical for assessing the necessity and appropriateness of the proposed medical interventions. For instance, if my patient was diagnosed with an eating disorder, I would expect that the reviewing physician was not only board-certified in psychiatry but that they also had clinical experience treating patients with eating disorders: anorexia, bulimia, binge eating disorder, and so forth.

Understanding the specific patient population and the unique challenges they present is a critical qualification. A peer should be familiar with the demographic, socioeconomic, and cultural factors that can influence patient care. This contextual knowledge helps in assessing the necessity and appropriateness of the proposed medical interventions, thus ensuring that the patient receives optimal care tailored to their individual needs.

The insurance company physician should be medically licensed in the same state as the practicing physician. State licensure ensures that the reviewing physician is familiar with the specific medical regulations, standards of care, and local healthcare environment. This familiarity is fundamental for making decisions that are not only medically sound but also compliant with local laws and guidelines.

Finally, the financial implications of the outcome of a peer-to-peer review should never be a consideration. Peer reviewers should never be compensated for or receive a "bonus" for treatment denials.

In summary, peer reviewers should be able to attest that they have thoroughly considered the substance of the case, have licensure and proper certification with a scope of knowledge that typically manages the medical condition, procedure, treatment or issues they have been asked to review, and that they possess current, relevant experience to render a determination about medical necessity. Unfortunately, prerequisite qualifications are not codified in law, so the definition of a "true" peer reviewer is debatable, and insurance companies continue to provide less than qualified peer reviewers to make critical, sometimes life-and-death decisions.

The AMA has been addressing peer review and other administrative harms for at least a half-dozen years. Several national insurers have announced plans to voluntarily reduce the number of services that require peer review and especially prior authorization. However, physicians report that health plans have made little progress honoring their commitments, and the administrative strain on healthcare professionals remains quite high. States have made some progress in passing laws to improve peer review, but more needs to be done.

24. Peer-to-Peer Review – Part 2

Insurance decisions that are internally inconsistent, ignore the "art of medicine," and do not consider the opinions of treating physicians are often made in bad faith.

Many physicians have shared their nightmare experiences with peer review and prior authorization as outlined in the previous essay. Prior authorization (PA) is a special type of peer review wherein the requested medical services, tests, and medications must first be approved by the health plan before patients can receive them. PA is different from "concurrent" peer review in which the patient is already receiving treatment and the medical necessity of further treatment is called into question.

Peer review, whether conducted prior to initial treatment or during treatment, is a Draconian practice that has upended physician autonomy and intruded in the doctor-patient relationship. The process has resulted in delayed treatment, treatment denied, and sometimes no treatment at all because physicians have been so worn down by the insurance machinery that they have given up trying to get the service approved, or have switched the patient to a therapy less preferred by the doctor but more preferred by the health plan because it costs less money. The results of this inane practice have caused unimaginable injustices for patients leading to severe morbidity and death in some instances.

A lawyer presented the case of a 47-year-old woman who complained of persistent leg pain even after 6 weeks of physical therapy. An orthopedic surgeon requested an MRI, which was denied by the insurance company. The decision was appealed, and it took 5 weeks for the company to reconsider approving the MRI, which revealed a sarcoma (bone cancer) on the patient's hip. It was necessary to amputate her leg, hip, and pelvis, along with chemotherapy. The patient was informed by the doctors that had she been seen a month sooner they would have treated her just with chemotherapy and no surgery. The lawyer made a plea to doctors, especially those "who are at the sunset of their careers," to fight insurance companies. It would be a "worthwhile coda to a worthy career," he opined.

The Case of Mr. A

Well…I took on an insurance company, and I wasn't even at the "sunset of my career" (I was in my mid-50s). The case revolved around a patient I'll call Mr. A. It is undisputed that he had Lyme disease (a tick-borne bacterial infection) with neurologic and ophthalmologic complications. Over the course of several years, the health plan had twice approved antibiotic therapy for Mr. A and twice denied it. Mr. A's physicians opined that the lack of timely treatment resulted in the deterioration of his eyesight and overall health.

Mr. A's attorney reached out to me in my capacity as an expert in health insurance. He asked me to review Mr. A's medical files. I wrote back that the inter-rater reliability of the health plan's medical directors, in terms of their decisions to approve and deny treatment benefits for Mr. A, was no better than a decision made by chance alone. Such arbitrary decision-making was unfair to patients such as Mr. A who depend on health plan medical directors to be consistent with each other and with their disease management guidelines. A 2011 audit of a sample of claims by the U.S. Government Accountability Office found that insurers reversed their initial decisions half the time, providing further evidence of inconsistent decision-making among health plans. (A more recent study by the Inspector General of the U.S. Department of Health and Human Services found that 73% of prior authorization denials for medications were approved on appeal.)

In addition, I told the attorney that utilization management guidelines should respect diverse medical views and should not be confined to narrowly interpreted scientific data. Experts generally agree that guidelines should be transparent to physicians and subscribers, free of conflicts of interest, and fully vetted by the medical community before they are implemented. They should be used to advance medical practice and aid clinical decision-making, not replace it. In Mr. A's case, however, the Lyme disease guidelines used by his health plan were very restrictive. They were based on controversial national guidelines modified by the health plan's internal medical policy committee, published online only, and silent as to the management of ophthalmologic complications.

Numb to Mr. A's Plight

In my report to Mr. A's lawyer, I discussed additional disturbing issues such as the ill-defined concept of "medical necessity," the confusing and cumbersome process for filing appeals, and the fact that Mr. A's health plan profited by avoiding costs associated with treatment had it been approved.

I criticized the conduct of the medical directors who worked for Mr. A's health plan. Physicians engaged in utilization review – so-called "physician advisors" – tend to become fixated on denying treatment, and they may become numb to the plight of patients such as Mr. A. As a former physician advisor myself, I know all too easily how some doctors become jaded in their decision-making, swallowing the insurance company's Kool-Aid.

I thought my arguments were airtight. I thought the case would be settled out of court. The health plan, however, refused to give in. It even went so far as to hire a former homicide prosecutor in the district attorney's office as its defense counsel. A trial date was set, and both parties agreed to a non-jury trial. Then came the proverbial shot heard round the world.

What Was He Thinking?

The health plan's chief medical officer (CMO) called my employer (a pharmaceutical company) to inform it that I was scheduled to testify. At the trial, the CMO testified that he informed my employer as a "courtesy," but my guess is he hoped my employer would get me to back down and forego testifying. Mr. A's attorney alleged a second count of bad faith on the part of the CMO for attempting to intimidate me from testifying. (The first count of bad faith was obviously the health plan's willy-nilly decision-making and arbitrary denial of medical benefits.)

Al parties were left to wonder what the CMO was thinking when he called my employer. His tip did cause my employer some concern, but after a discussion with company lawyers, I was cleared to testify.

The Trial Begins

When I finally had my day in court, I testified that I had indeed felt intimidated by the CMO's phone call. I thought, in retrospect, I might lose my job. Perhaps I had violated a company policy (I did not), or perhaps my employer might have second thoughts about my participation in the case. After all, my employer and the health plan had a business relationship.

Apparently, when the CMO placed the call, he was unaware that I had already received permission from my boss to be an expert witness in the case. When the CMO was asked by Mr. A's attorney if he had extended the same "courtesy" to other expert witnesses who testified on behalf of Mr. A, all the CMO could say was "no" – he never called the employers of the other doctors set to testify against the insurance company. I was the only expert witness the CMO singled out and threatened.

Attacked in Court

While I was on the witness stand, the health plan's medical directors attempted to stare me down. Its attorney attacked me relentlessly. He put *me* on trial, first by endeavoring to discredit my qualifications, and then by trying to impugn my integrity. He implied I was unfit to testify because one of my company's drugs was involved in product liability litigation. What shenanigans! The judge would have none of it. He said I was qualified as an expert, and I was cleared to proceed with my testimony.

The attorney and I got into a heated debate on the topic of evidence-based medicine. My position was that medical guidelines are not the holy grail – medicine is also an art – and that "cookbook medicine" is not always the right recipe for patients. I argued that the health plan's Lyme disease management guidelines could not be trusted for individual patients cared for by individual doctors. Even the national Lyme disease guidelines had a disclaimer to that effect, that there are clear distinctions between the health of a single patient and a population of patients.

In their article "The hazards of evidence-based medicine," Edward Livingston, MD, and Robert McNutt, MD, observed, "Variation in care is sometimes desirable. One patient's chronic illness is not another's, and treating all patients the same way would be clinical nonsense."

The Settlement

At the conclusion of the trial, the health plan's attorney moved for a summary dismissal of all charges. Apparently, the judge was unconvinced that the health plan had acted in bad faith, but he was certain that the motives of the CMO were not pure. The judge said he would consider the CMO's motives in his ruling, whereupon both defense and prosecution attorneys agreed to a settlement, and Mr. A was awarded compensation.

I was happy for Mr. A but disappointed that the court did not seem to recognize the injustices of utilization management. A health insurance company that arbitrarily disregards the recommendations of patients' physicians may not break any laws, but it is hardly acting in the best interest of patients.

The lawyer representing the patient with bone cancer came to a similar conclusion. He sued the insurance company and its utilization review subcontractor for malpractice – and lost. The lawyer wrote: "The courts said that while the story was tragic, there was no statute – and little case law – that said an insurance company had a duty of care to a patient. Doctors, nurses, podiatrists, dentists, hospitals, and medical practices all had a duty of care but not insurance companies."

I wonder? Do health plan medical directors who unthinkingly follow bottom-line oriented treatment algorithms to ration patient care have a reasonable basis for denying medical benefits to patients – and subsequently get away with it without any repercussions or consequences to their medical licenses? Medical practice, whether conducted at the bedside or in the corporate boardroom, is about integrating clinical expertise and the best external evidence for the welfare of patients. Anything less is bad faith.

REFLECTIONS

25. Reevaluating CEO Compensation in Health Care

The difficult task of balancing the scales of fairness.

Someone I've known since junior high school became a prominent physician and the head of a large nonprofit health system for 8½ years. During that time, he was compensated $45.6 million, averaging $4.56 million a year. He is wildly enthusiastic about the future of medicine, announcing on LinkedIn that he would be "unplugged" at an upcoming conference discussing the benefits of the blockbuster drug class of GLP-1s, initially marketed for diabetes and now gaining immense popularity for weight loss.

Heck, I'd be unplugged, too, for $45 million, but let's not stop there. In 2018, Bernard Tyson, then-CEO of nonprofit health care giant Kaiser Permanente, made nearly $18 million, making him the highest-paid nonprofit CEO in the nation. The previous year, the top 10 highest paid nonprofit health system executives each made $7 million or more.

And then there's the infamous case of Ralph de la Torre, MD, a brilliant Harvard-educated cardiovascular surgeon turned Chairman and CEO of the Steward Healthcare System, considered a "case study in executive greed." de la Torre made a fortune while his hospital chain collapsed, becoming one of the biggest hospital bankruptcies in decades. His activities have been under scrutiny by Congress and the Department of Justice, not least because hospital failures raised concerns about patient care and safety taking a back seat to financial gluttony – de la Torre owned yachts, jets, and luxurious homes, and he took lavish family vacations.

Steward paid at least $250 million to de la Torre and to his other companies during the four years he was the hospital chain's majority owner, which begs the question: what is equitable compensation for a hospital CEO? Mind you, some hospitals have fared better in the absence of CEO leadership, suggesting that the organizational structure, the strength of the management team, and the autonomy given to department heads and staff may play more important roles than the CEO.

The compensation of hospital and other healthcare CEOs is a hot topic, sparking debates among industry professionals, ethicists, and the general public. The same is true of CEOs in other industries, where in Seattle alone 2023 CEO compensation among Washington's largest public companies – Microsoft, T-Mobile, and Boeing – ranged from $32.7 million to $48.5 million. But of course, health care delivery is quite different than making software products, cell phones, and airplanes.

CEOs in health care make critical decisions that literally affect the lives of thousands of patients and employees, as well as the financial health of the organization. Leading a large healthcare system is an enormous responsibility, requiring exceptional skill, vision, and leadership. The argument here is that to attract and retain top talent capable of steering such complex entities, competitive compensation packages are necessary.

On the other hand, the staggering sums often associated with healthcare executive salaries can seem exorbitant, particularly in an industry fundamentally centered on care and compassion. Many argue that such high compensation is incongruous with the mission of health care, especially when frontline workers and essential staff often earn significantly less. The disparity between the salaries of healthcare executives and those of frontline healthcare workers, who are often overworked and underpaid, can be demoralizing and may impact the overall morale and effectiveness of the healthcare system. This discrepancy can foster a sense of injustice and contribute to ongoing issues of inequity within the healthcare system.

Moreover, there is the question of how these high salaries impact the overall cost of healthcare. Critics suggest that exorbitant executive compensation can drive up operational costs, potentially leading to higher costs for patients and insurers. Furthermore, there is concern that high compensation packages may incentivize CEOs to prioritize financial performance over patient care, leading to decisions that may not always align with the best interests of patients. In a system already criticized for its inefficiencies and high expenses, this is a concern that cannot be ignored.

Another important aspect to consider is the source of these funds. In many cases, healthcare systems are funded through public and private insurance, government programs, and patient payments. When a significant portion of these funds is allocated to executive salaries, it raises ethical questions about the allocation of resources in a system that is supposed to prioritize patient care and accessibility.

Transparency and accountability are key in addressing these concerns. Healthcare systems should ensure that executive compensation is tied to measurable improvements in patient care, operational efficiency, and community health outcomes. Additionally, there should be greater scrutiny of the potential conflicts of interest that arise from executives' relationships with pharmaceutical companies and other industry players. This is particularly pertinent in cases like my classmate's, where earnings from pharma consulting and speaking engagements further inflate compensation packages and potentially influence decision-making.

Ultimately, the debate about healthcare CEO compensation touches on broader issues of fairness, equity, and the true purpose of health care. While it's essential to reward talent and ensure effective leadership, there is a growing call for a more balanced approach that considers the welfare of all stakeholders, from patients and employees to the broader community. As we move forward, finding this balance will be central to shaping a healthcare system that is not only effective but also just and equitable.

No one has an answer to the question "how much is enough," but it raised many concerns among a group of academics writing in *Health Affairs*. They believed the answers could serve as guidelines for establishing fair and equitable pay for hospital CEOs, at least for nonprofit institutions. They felt that hospital boards in particular, as the final arbiters of CEO pay, should consider the following issues when deciding executive compensation:

- What should be the fundamental basis for CEO pay: size and complexity of the organization; organizational revenue; patient outcomes; community health; comparisons to for-profit corporate CEO pay?
- How should complexity or the degree of difficulty of the job be measured?
- Is there a maximum acceptable level of compensation? If bonuses are offered, what should they be based on?
- Should there be a norm established regarding the most equitable multiplier between CEO pay and general employee pay? Should there be a maximum?
- Should CEO pay and total compensation be reported and transparent for all individual hospitals as well as hospital systems?
- How much CEO pay is enough to ensure that hospitals are able to recruit effective leaders without further inflating the cost of health care, which is borne by all of us, or increasing wage disparities that harm communities?
- Revenue certainly places limits on what a hospital can pay. But when revenue is large, how much more should CEOs be rewarded for enhancing it further?

The *Health Affairs* authors concluded that nonprofit hospitals should be measured by the value they create – both business value and social value – and that all stakeholders should discuss the importance of aligning incentives to create real value in U.S. health care. Simply authorizing lavish executive compensation may leave hospitals in dire straits, with badly insufficient staffing and resources causing patient harm.

My classmate is now "chief visionary" of his own consulting firm and executive-in-residence at the world's largest venture capital investor in generative AI. His enthusiasm for the future of medicine, particularly around the GLP-1 drug class, is undiminished. But in an era where healthcare costs are skyrocketing and the disparity between executive compensation and frontline worker pay continues to widen, his earnings and credibility may receive greater attention than the promise of this new class of drugs.

26. Farewell Thoughts from a CEO

People are the most important asset of any company.

I have never been the CEO of a company. I never relished that role, assuming I was qualified. There's too much stress involved in being the CEO, with constant pressure to meet financial targets, make tough decisions, and be accountable for the success or failure of the organization. The demands on time and energy, along with the responsibility for employees' livelihoods and company reputation, can be overwhelming. I prefer roles where I can contribute meaningfully without bearing the immense burden that comes with being at the very top. Middle management is just fine with me (refer to essay 45).

But, if I were the CEO, I would want that role for, say, a dozen years. This timeframe would allow me to implement long-term strategies, see significant projects come to fruition, and foster a strong company culture. It would provide enough time to navigate the inevitable challenges and changes in the industry (obviously the healthcare industry), while also ensuring that I could leave a lasting positive impact on the organization. After those twelve years, I would likely step down to allow fresh leadership to bring new perspectives and ideas, ensuring the company's continued growth and innovation.

This paints a picture of a CEO I worked under toward the end of my career (he was not a physician). On his final day, he sent an email to all company employees. I'm sharing it here, slightly sanitized to preserve anonymity, because it's an inspiring account of the nature and purpose of work as well as a reminder that the most important asset of any company is the people who work for it.

Dear Fellow Team Members:

As I wrap up things and close out my time today as CEO, I wanted to take a minute and send you one final email and share three things: a thanks, a reflection, and a challenge.

First and foremost, thank you! It has been my honor, privilege and blessing to serve as the CEO since we formed the organization 12 years ago. I thank you all for your work, your dedication, your creativity and expertise, and your unwavering commitment to our mission and to those we have served. I thank you for the support you have given to me personally, for challenging me to be better, for your kind words through the years, and for the untold prayers and well wishes that you have poured onto me. Again – I say THANK YOU!

As I reflect on the last twelve years, and for the preceding twelve with one of our legacy programs, I have much pride in what we have done together. We have built something special here, something that I hope you are as proud of as I am. Through the years, we have served A LOT of people, and played an important part in helping others to live their best lives. That has been a noble undertaking, and again I hope you share the pride in our work.

We have also worked hard towards a culture that lives out the organizational values that we hold important. I am happy to have spent much time working to create an environment that challenges, supports and is rewarding and where all feel like we are truly a team. Though there are things now, and past decisions that not all liked or that not all would have made, I am proud that we have done what we have done with a commitment to being an organization of high integrity. Integrity is not assumed but rather earned, and can be fleeting if there is not a true commitment. I think we have been deeply committed to doing things with the highest level of integrity and I leave here proud of that.

Finally, I want to challenge all. First, as an organization…continue to focus on the mission and never waiver from its pursuit. As we continue to implement and grow new operations, and as future waves of change come from the state and elsewhere, I challenge the company to be guided by the North Star of our mission statement and never waiver. Continue to focus on excellence in all that is pursued and never cut corners and always do it "the right way."

More importantly, I challenge you all as individuals to be driven by your personal priorities. Know what is important to you in your lives and never settle and never compromise. Be driven by that every day and in every decision. Many have heard me talk about being driven by my faith, my family, and my relationships. I used our company to compliment that and not substitute for it, or to diminish it, or compromise it. I encourage you to do the same with whatever YOUR priorities are.

So, as I move on and pursue whatever is ahead in Chapter 2 for me while continuing to focus and be driven by those things important – my priorities, I wish our organization continued success, growth and impact on others and I wish each of you health, happiness, and success in using your priorities to LIVE YOUR BEST LIFE!

Sincerely,

[Name Withheld]

The CEO's letter effectively conveys a sense of closure, gratitude, and forward-looking optimism, leaving a lasting impression of a leader who truly cared about their team and the mission of the organization. What I find most fascinating is that the CEO's messages are universal and can be idealistically applied to any type of company in any industry.

The letter effectively communicates core values and leadership principles that transcend the healthcare industry. It highlights the importance of teamwork, integrity, and staying true to one's mission and personal priorities, which are applicable to any organization. The CEO's thoughtful farewell and inspiring message resonate with fundamental human and professional values, making the letter relevant and meaningful in any context.

27. Breaking Point: My Coworker's Resignation

A physician's resignation is often a response to burnout and moral injury, and it further depletes the workforce.

Despite the CEO's inspirational messages and deep care and commitment to the company's employees, as I described in the previous essay, if you read between the lines you will realize there were personnel casualties over time. There always are. But in health care, the thinning of the workforce is happening at an alarming rate.

A family medicine physician wrote that she burned out in her "dream job" just 18 months after completing her residency. Already down on herself and feeling like a failure, someone said to her, "If you leave, you're the reason the health care system is collapsing and there aren't enough doctors." Ultimately, however, the guilt this doctor felt about leaving wasn't enough to overcome the need to save herself.

A Harris poll of approximately 1000 physicians conducted online in late 2023 showed that more than half of participants (56%) said they've thought about either staying in medicine but no longer seeing patients, or leaving the field entirely.

A global survey by Elsevier Health revealed that 61% of medical and nursing students in the U.S. plan to work in non-patient-facing roles like public health, research, or business consulting. Alarmingly, 25% of medical students and 21% of nursing students reported considering quitting their studies altogether. Factors like well-being, moral injury, and long hours contribute to this sentiment.

Additional factors like interference from politicians, mental health concerns, work-life balance issues, and anticipated burnout are causing some medical students and residents to reconsider their career paths or avoid certain specialties and locations. According to the Association of American Medical Colleges, the U.S. will face a shortage of up to 86,000 physicians by 2036.

My coworker (a physician) announced her resignation in an email to the leadership team. She wrote:

To Whom It May Concern:

This letter is to inform you of my resignation. I have enjoyed many aspects of my time here, but it has become clear that it is no longer a good fit for me or my family. I remain dedicated to the population you serve and wish you all the best in moving forward.

My last day at work will be [in 2 months].

I will miss many of the kind, thoughtful folks who work here and so appreciate their dedication... I wish you all the best and hope for great future success.

Sincerely,

[Name withheld]

The architecture behind unprecedented physician turnover is likely multifactorial. Decreasing physician pay and increasing workload are major contributors to burnout and dissatisfaction among doctors. Many physicians feel they are not being fairly compensated, especially when factoring in inflation and the additional administrative burdens placed on them. 135 Medicare reimbursement rates for physicians have declined significantly over the past two decades, while patient care responsibilities have increased.

The COVID-19 pandemic exacerbated existing burnout issues, with a survey showing 63% of physicians experienced burnout in 2021, up from 38% in 2020. The intense stress and challenges faced during the pandemic have prompted some doctors to consider early retirement or career changes.

Employment models have shifted, with most physicians now working as employees rather than running private practices. This has led to a perceived loss of control and autonomy, as well as feelings of being undervalued by employers. Physicians may feel expendable in these arrangements.

There is also a lack of education for physicians on the business aspects of medicine, practice management, negotiation, and personal finance. This can contribute to feelings of disempowerment and an inability to advocate for fair compensation. Medical schools have traditionally been reluctant to incorporate business courses into their already demanding curricula.

The potential consequences of medical workers leaving the profession include worsening physician shortages, increasing gaps between specialties, and a decline in patient care quality. Efforts are needed at both systemic and individual levels to address these issues, such as advocating for physician well-being, reassessing practice structures, improving business and management education, and empowering physicians in negotiations.

The CEO tried to retain my coworker. This letter (above) was actually her second resignation. Her first occurred a month prior, but the CEO persuaded her to stay, so she rescinded it.

With her decision to leave now firm, we texted. She said:

"I got talked out of it [resigning] last time and my 3 days off last week were wonderful. I came back refreshed and a little more positive, but by yesterday I felt like a truck ran over me again. It's almost a physical illness how burned out and frustrated I am. I just can't keep doing this to myself and my family. I feel like I'm in a giant hole and can't see my way out. I needed an endpoint so I can see some light again. I feel like such a failure here."

I told my colleague that the company failed her and she shouldn't blame herself for not being able to stick it out. She is not a quitter, and her experience is not unique. Many healthcare workers are facing unprecedented challenges that lead to burnout, moral injury, and ultimately, the decision to resign.

Moral injury occurs when healthcare professionals are repeatedly exposed to situations that conflict with their ethical or moral beliefs. This can happen when they are unable to provide the level of care they believe is necessary due to system-wide constraints, such as understaffing, resource limitations, or administrative burdens.

My colleague's experience reflects this deeply. She describes feeling so burned out and frustrated that it feels like a physical illness, indicating an extreme sense of exhaustion and helplessness. Despite her resignation, she expresses continued dedication to the population served, highlighting the internal conflict between her professional commitment and the untenable work conditions.

Resignation is a last resort for healthcare workers who feel they cannot continue in their roles without compromising their health or personal lives. My colleague mentions that the job is no longer a good fit for her or her family, suggesting that the stress and demands of her role are affecting her personal life and well-being. Feeling like she is in a "giant hole" and needing an endpoint to "see some light again" points towards entrapment and the necessity of leaving to regain a sense of normalcy and health.

While the process of resigning, rescinding, and then resigning again can seem redundant, it can serve important purposes. It allows for thorough evaluation, provides a chance for organizational improvement, and ensures personal well-being is prioritized. However, I generally recommend gathering all necessary information and making a firm, one-time decision to resign. It promotes clarity, reduces stress, and prevents waffling or turning the resignation into a protracted negotiation.

Ultimately, the decision should be based on individual circumstances and the specific context of the physician's professional development. The most important factor is ensuring that the decision is well-considered and aligns with the physician's long-term goals and values.

28. I Was Quietly Fired Even Though I Complied

How long can you continue to work if you are shunned by your employer?

Less than a year into a new job as medical director at a health insurance company it surfaced that I had retained a small percentage of ownership in my former group practice. I never disclosed it to the company, and quite frankly, I didn't think it was necessary. However, in order to remain employed, I was required to sell my stake in the practice. The CEO informed me that he was being "kind" by letting me stay with the organization, and that undeclared conflicts of interest such as mine were grounds for immediate termination, as I might preferentially steer patients to that practice over others, and I stood to profit from that arrangement.

I divested my portion of the practice, but due to my initial lack of compliance (failure to report the conflict), I was quietly fired – allowed to stay with the company but demoted in position and moved to a basement office in a satellite location. Essentially, I was managed out, and I left the organization not long afterward.

What Is Quiet Firing?

"Quiet firing" refers to a situation where an employer subtly pushes an employee to resign rather than directly terminating their employment. This can be achieved through various means, such as gradually stripping away significant duties and responsibilities, excluding the employee from important meetings, projects, or decision-making processes, providing consistently negative feedback without basis or constructive criticism, denying promotions, raises, or professional development opportunities, assigning tasks that are excessively difficult or impossible to complete within given deadlines, and creating a work environment that is uncomfortable or hostile, making the employee feel unwelcome.

Physicians might be quietly fired due to failure to meet evolving productivity targets, disagreements with administrative decisions, or persistent clashes with colleagues or superiors. Furthermore, changes in hospital policies, restructuring, or a shift toward more profitable specialties can result in decreased support, undesirable shifts, or reduced responsibilities, making the work environment untenable for the physician. This approach allows institutions to avoid potential legal disputes and public backlash while gradually encouraging the physician to leave voluntarily.

A quiet firing can have significant professional and personal implications. Physicians may find it challenging to secure new positions if they leave their current role under such circumstances. Negative performance reviews and lack of recent achievements can impact their professional reputation. A physician experiencing quiet firing might be distracted or demoralized, which could negatively affect their ability to provide high-quality patient care.

The stress and uncertainty associated with quiet firing can lead to burnout, anxiety, and other mental health issues. Additionally, physicians need to ensure they are complying with medical and ethical standards despite the difficult work environment. Quiet firing tactics could indirectly pressure them to compromise on these standards. Being quietly fired can strain relationships with colleagues and patients, which are crucial for successful medical practice.

One physician described his quiet firing this way: "…often subtle but firm pressure, manipulative changes, and general discomfort designed to make you want to leave. It is a cold, calculating, passive-aggressive business approach to help guide a person away from continued employment. At first, you may think it is a small event that you simply overlooked, but those events quickly add up and escalate.

Your work is never good enough, your approach is overlooked, you might even be ignored, and over time you wonder how you could even improve. Could this truly be your problem, or is something else at play here? Eventually, time, examples, and intuition tell you something is not right."

What You Should Do If You Are Being Quietly Fired

Physicians who feel they are being quietly fired can take several steps to address the situation. They should keep detailed records of changes in responsibilities, performance reviews, and any communication that might indicate quiet firing. Attempting to have open and honest conversations with supervisors or HR about their concerns and seeking feedback is important. Engaging with professional organizations, mentors, or legal counsel can help them understand their rights and options.

I never sought legal advice on the matter, but my research has led me to believe that there is no definitive answer to whether a physician employed by a health insurance company can retain partial ownership of an in-network group practice. I imagine I should have consulted a legal expert before starting the job to ensure I was in full compliance with all relevant laws and company policies. Better yet, I should have declared the conflict upfront whether or not I believed it was relevant. This is what virtually all corporate compliance officers will advise new or potential hires, and it would be prudent to seek out legal advice of your own if you suspect quiet firing.

If you try to hang on as you are being quietly fired, be prepared to be treated poorly while seeking affirmation and answers from colleagues. You must prioritize your mental and physical health, take a step back, and view the situation objectively. Would you advise a family member to keep enduring, taking punishment, and asking for more? Understanding the dynamics of quiet firing and its implications can help you navigate the situation more effectively by knowing when to leave and protecting your career and well-being.

I knew it was time leave within a few short months after the CEO confronted me. My responsibilities gradually shifted and became mundane. My role was diminished and no longer aligned with my skills and interests. The isolation excluded me from important meetings and decisions. My efforts were being deliberately overlooked. I realized my professional development would be limited and there would be no opportunity for career advancement.

I looked for new employment, and I timed my exit with a new job, protecting my career by telling my new employer that my old job was no longer a good fit. I was careful not to “trash” my former company on the way out. I wasn’t worried about a relatively short stint appearing on my CV and what that might signal. The average medical director stays at their job for a few years, and physicians in full-time corporate practice also seem to change jobs quickly. In my experience – and I believe HR personnel would attest to this – the gold watch is a relic of the past.

29. When EMS "Grandstanding" Almost Cost a Life

A display of ignorance, arrogance, and mistrust in emergency medical care.

A colleague texted me the following story.

"Hectic night last night [at a public event]. At the end of the show, they called for a doctor or any medical professional to aid in the care of someone who passed out. Naturally, I responded...a young guy 23 years old passed out, dehydrated, easily woke up, complained of chest pain intermittently, and passed out on me 3 more times. Weak and bradycardic pulses but never lost a pulse. I kept calling out for EMS [emergency medical services], cardiac monitor, AED [automated external defibrillator], etc.

When EMS finally arrived, I told them I need a glucose check, cardiac monitor/EKG, IV with one liter IV fluid bolus, etc. They were a little offended with me spouting off orders, said they would do all that in the ambulance, once we moved him out of the grand stand. I kept arguing not to move him until I felt comfortable with his cardiac rhythm, glucose check, and oxygen in place.

They overruled me, placed him on a backboard, and we all carried him down the steps when he passed out again, and then I lost my shit. Thankfully, he didn't lose a pulse, we got him into the ambulance, and I went off on them...telling them to do immediately what I asked them to do previously. Then I told them to turn on the sirens and drive fast to ER.

A few minutes later, several people found me, thanked me, and asked me what went wrong (everything) and what could be done better?"

I texted my colleague back and wrote: "You are double-board certified [internal medicine and pediatrics] with 20+ years of experience. And EMS training is how long? Unbelievable story of ignorance, arrogance, and mistrust."

1. **Ignorance**: There may have been a lack of understanding or awareness on the part of the EMS team regarding the urgency of the patient's condition and the rationale behind my colleague's requests. Ensuring that all medical professionals involved in emergency care are well-informed and up-to-date on best practices is essential.
2. **Arrogance**: The EMS team's reluctance to follow my colleague's advice and their decision to prioritize their standard protocols over the immediate concerns of a highly trained medical professional could be seen as a display of arrogance. This attitude can hinder effective teamwork and compromise patient care.
3. **Mistrust**: The situation also reflects a possible mistrust between professionals with different levels and types of training. Trust is crucial in emergency settings, where quick, coordinated action by many people is necessary.

I began to further ponder the question: What could have been done better? While everything may have seemed to go wrong, a few key takeaways and suggestions for improvement came to mind:

1. **Communication and Teamwork**: It is crucial to establish clear and respectful communication with EMS personnel. A quick briefing on roles and expectations could prevent misunderstandings. I understand that maintaining composure in an emergency is difficult, but perhaps my colleague could have calmly explained his rationale for specific requests, emphasizing the patient's immediate needs. EMS personnel definitely need to lower their guard and follow his commands.

2. **On-Site Assessment and Stabilization**: Suggestions to obtain a glucose check, cardiac monitor, and IV fluids on-site were valid given the patient's condition. This highlights the importance of having essential equipment readily available at public events, especially AEDs to treat sudden cardiac arrest. Event organizers could ensure better preparedness by having medical kits, including glucose meters and portable cardiac monitors, on hand.
3. **Protocol and Training**: EMS teams typically follow strict protocols, which they might prioritize over ad-hoc instructions. It might be beneficial to advocate for training sessions where medical professionals and EMS teams can collaborate and understand each other's protocols and priorities better. While it might seem like a tall order to bring disparate individuals together in large cities, it is quite possible to accomplish this in small, rural communities where my colleague practices.
4. **Patient Safety During Transport**: My colleague's concern about moving the patient before stabilization is valid. Emphasizing the importance of patient safety during transport to EMS might help them understand the gravity of the situation. The Emergency Medical Treatment and Labor Act (EMTALA) embodies the principle of stabilization over transportation.
5. **Post-Incident Review**: Conducting a debriefing session with EMS and event organizers can help identify what went wrong and how to improve future responses. This can include reviewing the availability of medical equipment, communication strategies, and response protocols.

Above all, let's not forget civility. Although the public were grateful for my colleague's actions, the EMS team never thanked him for his dedication and quick thinking in a critical situation.

30. Vexing Psychiatric Patients – Part 1

Vexing patients are defined along different dimensions and by different criteria.

I have more that 40 years of psychiatric experience. As you can imagine, I have treated many difficult patients. Here are some of the more vexing ones:

- A young man repeatedly hammered nails into his calf muscle. He cut off the heads of the nails to make it more difficult for the surgeons to remove them.
- An elderly man had severe depression and unremitting obsessions depicting family members engaged in various lewd sex acts. No matter how hard he tried, he could not vanquish the disturbing images from his mind.
- A female nurse presented with septic arthritis (infection) of the knee. She was suspected of producing this infection and others.
- A pyromaniac was involuntarily committed for psychiatric treatment. He had a history of targeting and setting fire to his therapists' homes. I feared I would be next.
- A teenager impulsively overdosed on Tylenol following a breakup with her boyfriend. She was unaware that Tylenol could cause liver damage, and she died awaiting a liver transplant.
- A young woman had received a significant amount of antipsychotic medication. She developed stiff muscles, profuse sweating, mental status changes, hyperthermia, and other abnormal vital signs indicative of neuroleptic malignant syndrome (NMS). The syndrome was virtually unknown at the time (1980), and there was no established treatment.
- A middle-aged woman had a history of schizophrenia and long-term treatment with antipsychotic medication that caused

severe, uncontrollable movements (tardive dyskinesia). Her excessive movements led to myoglobinuric renal failure (due to over-exertion) and death.

- A young man shared the same delusions as his twin brother (folie à deux). Neither brother could be dissuaded from their false beliefs.
- An elderly African American woman had lived the past quarter century with the belief that she had been "rooted" (cursed or hexed through supernatural means), resulting in continuous physical suffering without a medical explanation (somatic delusions).

This list represents the tip of the iceberg of patients I found interesting yet difficult to treat. Determining whether a psychiatric patient should be considered "vexing" involves evaluating several interrelated factors that encompass the complexity, severity, and manageability of their condition.

Patients with severe and persistent symptoms that resist standard treatments often fall into this category, particularly when these symptoms are chronic and show little improvement despite multiple interventions. Treatment resistance has become a significant marker, as patients who do not respond to conventional therapies, including medications and psychotherapy, may necessitate exploring more intensive, experimental, or combination treatments, which can be resource-intensive and carry additional risks.

The presence of comorbid conditions further complicates diagnosis and treatment; for example, patients with both a severe mental illness and a substance use disorder may require integrated care approaches and present with more unpredictable treatment courses. Behavioral challenges also play a crucial role, with patients exhibiting disruptive behaviors or posing risks to themselves or others often considered vexing. This includes those with high impulsivity, aggression, self-harm tendencies, or non-compliance with treatment plans. Interpersonal difficulties, such as those seen in patients with borderline personality disorder, can lead to frequent crises, emotional volatility, and challenges in maintaining a stable and effective therapeutic alliance.

High utilization of healthcare resources is another indicator, with patients frequently requiring hospitalizations, emergency room visits, and intensive outpatient services often demanding a disproportionate amount of time, effort, and resources from the healthcare system. Patients at high risk of self-harm or suicide, or those who may harm others, require constant monitoring and intervention, adding to the complexity of their care. Ensuring their safety often involves multidisciplinary approaches and can lead to significant emotional and professional stress for healthcare providers.

The pyromaniac (above) challenged my stress tolerance for obvious reasons. Suicidal patients did as well. No one wants a suicide on their record. Apart from the tragedy of the event and the distress caused to loved ones, there is a belief among many medical professionals that a psychiatrist should never lose a patient. The truth is: it is sometimes unavoidable, as is homicide. One of my colleagues evaluated a patient in a "crisis center." The patient was discharged without being hospitalized. The following day the patient killed a family member. My colleague was devastated.

Another colleague, a co-resident, faced enormous pressure while treating a young woman who was chronically suicidal. She had, in fact, jumped in front of a train and miraculously survived. My colleague feared she would do it again, so he adopted a "soft" approach in therapy with her. Our supervisor observed this dynamic and offered a candid, albeit controversial, piece of advice: "The difference between you and me is that you're afraid of that damn train and I'm not." This statement highlighted a stark contrast in perspectives on managing high-risk patients and illustrated the delicate balance between empathy and effective clinical intervention. The supervisor was essentially suggesting that the patient's quality of life was so poor that she might be better off dead, rather than continuing to live in such a state.

This perspective was intended to provoke a deeper reflection on the therapeutic approach, emphasizing that while empathy is crucial, it must be coupled with a realistic and sometimes tough evaluation of the patient's overall well-being. This approach encourages patients to confront and manage their behaviors more effectively, rather than merely providing comfort without addressing the underlying issues.

This experience serves as a valuable reminder of the importance of maintaining professional boundaries and utilizing a balanced approach in therapy – one that combines compassion with firm, evidence-based interventions, and a realistic assessment of the patient's quality of life. It also signifies that impairment in daily functioning, including the inability to maintain employment, relationships, or self-care, makes management more complex. Such patients may need comprehensive support that goes beyond standard psychiatric care, including social services and community support. These factors provide a framework for understanding why certain psychiatric patients may be considered particularly vexing, often requiring a high degree of expertise, multidisciplinary collaboration, and innovative treatment strategies to manage them effectively.

31. Vexing Psychiatric Patients – Part 2

Can psychiatric diagnoses predict adults – and children – who are difficult to treat?

Psychiatric practice involves managing a wide array of complex and challenging cases, but certain patient profiles can be particularly vexing due to the nature of their conditions and the difficulties inherent in their treatment. Compared with the previous essay, which discussed problematic patients phenomenologically, this essay focuses on psychiatric diagnoses as predictors of difficulty.

One such group includes individuals with borderline personality disorder (BPD). Patients with BPD often present with intense emotional instability, fear of abandonment, and impulsive behaviors, which can lead to frequent crises and self-harm. Their relationships, including those with healthcare providers, can be tumultuous, marked by idealization and devaluation, which makes establishing and maintaining a therapeutic alliance particularly challenging. The erratic nature of their symptoms and the high risk of self-injury or suicidal behavior require constant vigilance and can strain the resources of mental health professionals.

Another challenging group consists of patients with treatment-resistant depression, affecting approximately 30% of persons receiving antidepressant treatment in research settings and between 6 and 55% in "real world" practice. These individuals have typically undergone multiple therapeutic interventions, including various medications and psychotherapies, with little to no improvement. The persistent nature of their depressive symptoms can lead to hopelessness and despair, not only for the patients but also for the clinicians treating them. The lack of response to conventional treatments necessitates the exploration of more intensive and often experimental approaches, such as electroconvulsive therapy (ECT) or ketamine infusions, which come with their own risks and ethical considerations.

Patients with severe, chronic schizophrenia also represent a vexing population to treat. The enduring nature of their psychotic symptoms, such as delusions and hallucinations, coupled with cognitive impairments and "negative" symptoms like apathy and social withdrawal, can make it difficult to achieve meaningful improvements in their quality of life. These patients often require long-term, multifaceted treatment plans that combine medication, psychosocial interventions, and community support services. The complexity and chronicity of schizophrenia can lead to frequent hospitalizations and a high burden of care, which can be daunting for both patients and healthcare providers.

Lastly, individuals with substance use disorders pose unique and difficult challenges. The interplay between addiction and mental illness can complicate diagnosis and treatment, as substance use can exacerbate psychiatric symptoms and vice versa. These patients often exhibit non-compliance with treatment, high rates of relapse, and a tendency to engage in risky behaviors, which can undermine therapeutic efforts and lead to repeated crises and hospitalizations.

Thus, while all psychiatric patients deserve compassionate and comprehensive care, those with personality disorders, treatment-resistant depression, severe and persistent mental illnesses such as schizophrenia, and comorbid substance use disorders often present as the most vexing. Their conditions require a high degree of clinical expertise, patience, and resourcefulness to manage them effectively, highlighting the need for ongoing research, interdisciplinary collaboration, and innovative treatment approaches in the field of psychiatry.

At this juncture, it is relevant to ask about the children of individuals diagnosed with severe mental disorders. A 2024 population-based register study done in Sweden sheds light. Associations were examined between six psychiatric diagnoses in parents and a broad range of psychiatric and nonpsychiatric outcomes in their offspring.

The six diagnoses consisted of schizophrenia, bipolar disorder, depression, anxiety, alcohol-related disorder, and other substance use disorder.

Not surprisingly, children with parents who had one of the six psychiatric diagnoses were more likely to have a psychiatric diagnosis themselves when compare to the offspring of parents without a psychiatric diagnosis. The probabilities were consistent and ranged from 22% (of children exposed to parental depression) to 25% (of children exposed to parental drug-related disorders). However, children who had parents with psychiatric diagnoses were not necessarily diagnosed with the same or related psychiatric conditions as their parents, suggesting that intergenerational transmission of parenteral psychiatric disorders is largely "transdiagnostic."

The outcomes for children of parents with major psychiatric disorders can be influenced by various factors, including the type and severity of the parent's disorder, the presence of supportive family and social networks, and access to mental health care and other resources. These children are at an increased risk for developing psychiatric conditions themselves, due to both genetic predispositions and environmental influences. This includes a higher likelihood of experiencing mood disorders, anxiety disorders, and other mental health issues.

Emotionally and behaviorally, these children may exhibit a range of problems, such as increased anxiety, depression, conduct issues, and difficulties with emotional regulation. These challenges often stem from the stress and instability associated with living with a parent who has a major psychiatric disorder. Academically, difficulties are common, often due to a combination of cognitive, emotional, and behavioral challenges. Children may struggle with attention, concentration, and motivation, which can impact their performance in school.

Social relationships can also be more difficult for these children. They might experience social isolation, bullying, or difficulties in peer relationships due to the stigma associated with their parent's condition or their own behavioral issues. The quality of the parent-child relationship can be significantly affected as well. Children may experience inconsistent parenting, emotional unavailability, or even neglect if the parent's psychiatric condition is severe. Conversely, some children may take on caregiving roles, leading to increased stress and a sense of burden.

However, not all outcomes are negative. Many children demonstrate remarkable resilience, particularly when protective factors are present. These can include a stable and supportive relationship with another caregiver or family member, access to mental health services, involvement in supportive educational environments, and the presence of strong social support networks.

Early intervention and ongoing support are crucial in mitigating negative outcomes. This can include counseling and therapy for the child, parenting support and education for the parent, and coordination with schools to provide academic and social support. Community resources and support groups can also play a vital role in providing stability and assistance.

It is incumbent on clinicians working with adult patients who have psychiatric diagnoses to consider a wide range of diagnostic and behavioral outcomes in their children. Likewise, providers beyond mental health settings, e.g., criminal justice and educational and social services, need to consider clients' broader psychiatric and family history. While children of parents with major psychiatric disorders face increased risks for a range of challenges, the presence of supportive interventions and protective factors can significantly improve their outcomes and help them lead fulfilling lives.

32. Balancing Diagnosis and Symptomatic Treatment

To diagnose or not to diagnose – that *is the question!*

For many patients with lower back pain, anti-inflammatory medication and physical therapy alone will make a huge difference and are likely to be the only treatment needed. Extensive workups are not advised unless pain persists for more than several weeks.

Dozens of viruses (and even some bacteria) can cause upper respiratory symptoms such as a runny nose, cough, sore throat, and low-grade fever. Doctors don't typically test for any of them (COVID being an important exception) because knowing which bug is to blame won't change treatment; common upper-respiratory infections are short-lived and generally not harmful to your health.

Other conditions, however, rely heavily on an exact diagnosis for treatment. Cancer, for example, is defined by anatomic origin, genetic data (if available), degree of spread, and many other factors. These details inform the diagnosis, which will then shape the kind of treatment offered as well as the prognosis.

In psychiatry, I've witnessed an opposite approach to treatment that relies on treating the patient's symptoms rather than the underlying condition(s). This type of "shotgun" therapy is reflected in the growth of polypharmacy over the past few decades. Polypharmacy involves a combination of medications from different classes, such as antidepressants, antipsychotics, mood stabilizers, and anxiolytics, intended to target different aspects of a patient's symptoms. I've always considered polypharmacy a sign that the prescriber is not sure about the patient's diagnosis.

I was taught to always make a diagnosis first, because treatment follows from a correct diagnosis, and an incorrect diagnosis could lead to the wrong treatment including drug interactions, side effects, and medication nonadherence. The doctrine I preach to trainees is that establishing an accurate diagnosis is a fundamental principle in psychiatry, as well as in all areas of medicine. The rationale behind this approach is that treatment should be tailored to address the specific underlying condition – not the symptoms – ensuring that the interventions are appropriate and effective.

Here are a few key points I highlight to underscore the importance of making a correct diagnosis before initiating treatment:

1. **Targeted Treatment**: An accurate diagnosis allows for the selection of treatments that are specifically effective for that condition, whether they are pharmacological, psychotherapeutic, or a combination of both.
2. **Avoiding Harm**: Incorrect diagnosis can lead to inappropriate treatment, which may not only be ineffective but also potentially harmful. For example, prescribing an antidepressant for someone with bipolar depression mistakenly diagnosed with major depressive disorder could trigger a manic episode.
3. **Resource Utilization**: Accurate diagnosis helps in the efficient use of healthcare resources, ensuring that patients receive the most appropriate and cost-effective care.
4. **Patient Trust:** Patients may perceive that not pursuing a detailed diagnosis means that their doctor isn't concerned or that something is being missed. On the other hand, a detailed and specific diagnosis is validating, and it may help patients educate themselves about their condition or join a support community.
5. **Compliance**: A correct diagnosis increases a patient's understanding of their condition and usually leads to better compliance with treatment.
6. **Comprehensive Care**: Diagnosis allows for a holistic approach to patient care, addressing not only the primary condition but also any comorbidities that may be present.

But I also realize that diagnoses can be elusive, and deciding whether to continue searching for one, even after a tentative diagnosis has been made, or to shift focus to symptomatic treatment, can be quite baffling. There are several factors to consider in making this decision.

If a patient develops new symptoms or if existing symptoms worsen, it may be necessary to investigate further. Similarly, if the patient does not respond to treatment as usual, this could indicate an underlying cause that requires more in-depth examination. The presence of "red flags," such as unexplained weight loss, persistent fever, or other alarming signs, should also prompt further diagnostic efforts. Additionally, if the patient is particularly anxious about their symptoms or strongly disagrees with it, it may be beneficial to continue investigating or seek a second opinion. If there is a reasonable possibility that the symptoms are indeed due to another condition, further diagnostic efforts may be justified.

On the other hand, for chronic conditions where extensive diagnostic efforts have already been made without yielding a clear diagnosis, it may be more beneficial to focus on managing symptoms. If ongoing diagnostic procedures are causing significant stress, discomfort, or impacting the patient's quality of life, shifting to symptomatic treatment may be more appropriate. This is particularly relevant in elderly patients or those with multiple comorbidities, where the risks and burdens of extensive diagnostic procedures may outweigh the potential benefits. If the patient prefers to focus on symptom management rather than further diagnostic testing, their wishes should be respected. Additionally, if the symptoms are stable and not significantly impacting the patient's daily life, managing them symptomatically may be reasonable.

Whether or not there is a detailed diagnosis, it is important to explore how patients' symptoms affect how they function and feel, both physically and emotionally. In fact, sometimes putting aside the search for a diagnosis allows more time for having these important conversations and helps both physician and patient to gain insight into treatment goals.

Balancing the two approaches – diagnosing and managing symptoms – involves regular reassessment of the patient's condition and being open to revisiting the diagnostic process if new information arises. Engaging the patient in the decision-making process ensures that their values and preferences are considered. Involving other healthcare professionals, such as specialists, can provide additional perspectives and expertise. Ultimately, the decision should be individualized, taking into account the specific circumstances of the patient, the potential benefits and risks of further diagnostic testing, and the overall goals of care.

While I have not changed my fundamental position over the years, i.e., diagnosis is all-important, I now think of it as one step in the evaluation and treatment process, not necessarily the first (or only). Pausing on a search for a detailed diagnosis isn't necessarily giving up, being lazy, or practicing sloppy medicine. Sometimes taking the time to explore the physical and emotional impact of symptoms, instead of being narrowly focused on diagnosis alone, will likely be more helpful to both patients and physicians in the long run.

33. The Importance of Lived Experience in Medicine

Embracing patients' narratives leads to better care.

Lived experience in medicine refers to the insights and understandings that patients gain through their personal journeys with illness, treatment, and healthcare systems. This concept emphasizes the subjective, personal, and often emotional aspects of dealing with health conditions, which can be as essential as clinical knowledge in providing holistic care. Understanding lived experiences can enhance empathy among healthcare providers, improve patient care, and lead to more patient-centered approaches in medicine. None of the essays in this book could have been written without the awareness of my patients' narratives and their trusted exchanges with me as their doctor.

A prime example of lived experience in medicine is the narrative of chronic illness patients. Individuals with conditions such as diabetes, rheumatoid arthritis, or multiple sclerosis navigate a daily landscape of symptom management, medication adherence, and lifestyle adjustments. Their stories reveal the ongoing challenges and adaptations required to maintain quality of life. For instance, a patient with diabetes might describe the constant vigilance needed to monitor blood sugar levels, the impact on their social life, and the emotional toll of managing a lifelong condition. These insights can guide healthcare providers to offer more appropriate support and resources, recognizing the full spectrum of the patient's daily struggles and triumphs.

Another significant area where lived experience plays a crucial role is in mental health. Patients with depression, anxiety, or bipolar disorder often articulate experiences that go beyond clinical symptoms, encompassing feelings of isolation, stigma, and the personal journey towards finding effective treatment. A person with depression might share how the condition affects their motivation, relationships, and self-perception, offering a depth of understanding that clinical descriptions alone cannot capture. These personal accounts can help mental health professionals tailor interventions that acknowledge the patient's unique context and emotional landscape, fostering a more compassionate and effective therapeutic environment.

Lived experience is also vital in understanding the impact of terminal illness. Patients facing end-of-life issues provide invaluable perspectives on what truly matters in their remaining time. Their experiences can highlight the importance of palliative care, advance directives, and the need for emotional and spiritual support. For example, a patient with advanced cancer might express a desire for pain management, the significance of spending time with loved ones, and the need for clear communication about their prognosis. These insights can inform healthcare providers how to approach end-of-life care, ensuring it aligns with the patient's values and wishes.

Moreover, the lived experiences of caregivers offer another layer of understanding in medicine. Family members and friends who support patients through illness provide a unique viewpoint on the emotional and practical challenges of caregiving. They often navigate complex healthcare systems, manage medications, and provide emotional support, all while balancing their own lives. A caregiver's account can illuminate the need for better support systems, respite care, and resources that acknowledge their critical role in the patient's health journey.

Incorporating lived experiences into medical practice requires active listening and empathy from healthcare providers. It means valuing the patient's voice as a key component of their care and recognizing that their stories can inform and improve medical practice. By integrating these personal narratives, health care can become more responsive, compassionate, and effective, ultimately leading to better health outcomes and patient satisfaction.

Lived experience in medicine enriches the understanding of health and illness beyond clinical symptoms and treatments. People with lived experience know things that clinicians and scientists do not. A simple statement can move the needle on healthcare innovation across multiple domains, from patient safety to devices to drug development to clinical trial recruitment (refer to essay 11).

In patient safety, for example, individuals with lived experience can identify potential risks and hazards that may not be apparent to healthcare providers. Their feedback can lead to the development of safer protocols and environments that better accommodate patient needs. In the realm of medical devices, patient input can guide the design process to ensure that products are user-friendly and truly meet the needs of those who will use them. For instance, a diabetic patient's experience with insulin pumps can provide essential feedback on usability and comfort, leading to more effective and accessible devices.

In drug development, patients can offer perspectives on side effects and quality-of-life issues that go beyond what is captured in clinical trials. Their experiences can help prioritize which drug attributes matter most, ensuring that new treatments not only extend life but also improve its quality. Furthermore, in clinical trial recruitment, understanding the barriers and motivators from a patient's point of view can enhance enrollment strategies, making trials more inclusive and representative of diverse populations.

By recognizing and integrating the knowledge gained from lived experiences, health care can become more patient-centered, innovative, and effective. This approach can lead to the development of solutions that are not only clinically sound but also practically relevant and compassionate, ultimately improving outcomes and satisfaction for patients. Because lived experiences encompass the personal, emotional, and social dimensions of healthcare, providing a more comprehensive view of what patients endure, healthcare providers can enhance their empathy and improve patient care by valuing and integrating these experiences in their practice.

34. Recommended Books and Works on Lived Experience

Diverse and multifaceted perspectives on lived experiences offer readers a blend of personal stories and theoretical insights, enriching their comprehension of the complexities of life and human experience.

To gain a deeper understanding of "lived experience" in medicine, several compelling books and works stand out for their insightful narratives and thoughtful reflections. *The Emperor of All Maladies: A Biography of Cancer* by Siddhartha Mukherjee, MD, is a masterful blend of history, science, and personal stories that provides a comprehensive look at cancer through the eyes of both patients and physicians. Mukherjee's narrative brings to life the human aspects of battling cancer, highlighting the resilience and challenges faced by those affected. He insightfully observes: "Medicine…begins with storytelling. Patients tell stories to describe illness; doctors tell stories to understand it. Science tells its own story to explain diseases…"

Another essential read is *Being Mortal: Medicine and What Matters in the End* by Atul Gawande, MD. Gawande, a surgeon, tackles the complexities of aging and end-of-life care with empathy and clarity, using real-life stories to illuminate the often-overlooked experiences of patients and their families. His exploration of how the medical system handles mortality is both enlightening and thought-provoking, emphasizing the importance of understanding patient perspectives.

For a more patient-centered viewpoint, *When Breath Becomes Air* by Paul Kalanithi, MD, is a poignant memoir by a neurosurgeon diagnosed with terminal lung cancer. Kalanithi's reflections on his transition from doctor to patient provide a powerful and intimate look at the lived experience of illness, mortality, and the search for meaning. Kalanithi's career as a surgeon and writer was tragically cut short at age 37. His book was published posthumously in 2016, a year after his death.

The Immortal Life of Henrietta Lacks by Rebecca Skloot details the story of Henrietta Lacks, whose cancer cells were taken without her knowledge and used for groundbreaking medical research (refer to essay 12). Skloot weaves together scientific discovery with the personal and ethical implications for Lacks' family, offering a profound examination of the intersection between medical progress and individual lives.

For those interested in mental health, *An Unquiet Mind: A Memoir of Moods and Madness* by Kay Redfield Jamison, PhD, provides an insider's perspective on living with bipolar disorder. As both a clinical psychologist and a patient, Jamison's dual perspective enriches the narrative, offering valuable insights into the experience and treatment of mental illness.

To fully grasp the multifaceted concept of "lived experience," it is also beneficial to explore works spanning philosophy, sociology, feminist theory, and critical race studies. These disciplines offer diverse perspectives on how individuals perceive, interpret, and navigate their realities. This is essential reading for students in narrative medicine programs.

Diving into phenomenology, Edmund Husserl's *Ideas: General Introduction to Pure Phenomenology* lays the groundwork for understanding consciousness from a first-person perspective. Maurice Merleau-Ponty's *Phenomenology of Perception* further explores how our bodily existence shapes our experiences, emphasizing the intertwined nature of perception and embodiment. Additionally, Martin Heidegger's *Being and Time* delves deep into the structures of existence, offering insights into the temporal and contextual aspects of lived experience.

In the realm of sociology, Erving Goffman's *The Presentation of Self in Everyday Life* examines the intricacies of social interactions, highlighting how individuals curate their identities in various contexts. Pierre Bourdieu's *Distinction: A Social Critique of the Judgement of Taste* provides an undeniable analysis of how cultural capital and social stratification influence personal experiences and perceptions.

Simone de Beauvoir's seminal work, *The Second Sex*, offers a tour de force of women's lived experiences within patriarchal structures. Frantz Fanon's *Black Skin, White Masks* delves into the psychological impacts of colonialism and racism on Black individuals, revealing the complexities of identity formation. Bell Hooks' *Feminist Theory: From Margin to Center* challenges mainstream feminist discourse by centering the experiences of marginalized women, thus broadening the understanding of lived realities.

Ta-Nehisi Coates' *Between the World and Me* presents a poignant narrative on the Black American experience, weaving personal anecdotes with broader socio-political commentary. *How Dare We! Write*, a volume edited by Sherry Quan Lee, calls out to people of color everywhere, demonstrating that lived experiences can unearth the roots of our heritage and help us stand up to traditions that silence us.

Psychiatrist Bessel van der Kolk's *The Body Keeps the Score* is an essential read that bridges the gap between lived experience and the body's response to trauma. This book vividly portrays how our bodies carry the imprints of our experiences, making it a fascinating account of the physical manifestations of lived experiences.

Engaging with these works provides a comprehensive lens through which to appreciate the depth and diversity of lived experiences across different contexts and identities. Collectively they underscore the importance of integrating lived experiences into the understanding of health and medicine.

35. You Can't Outrun a Memory

The inevitability of memory represents inescapable echoes of our past lives.

The phrase "you can't outrun a memory" does not have a well-documented origin or attribution to a specific author or historical figure. It appears to be a piece of folk wisdom or a saying that has evolved over time, encapsulating a common human experience. The concept it expresses, i.e., memories, especially those that are emotionally charged, cannot simply be left behind, resonates widely across cultures and contexts, which may explain its prevalence in various forms of literature, music, and colloquial speech.

While the exact origin remains unclear, the sentiment behind the phrase is echoed in many works of literature and art throughout history. For example, themes of inescapable memories and the enduring impact of the past are common in classical literature, such as in the works of Shakespeare, who often explored the persistence of guilt, regret, and unresolved emotions.

"The Scream," painted by Norwegian artist Edvard Munch in 1893, is iconic for its powerful depiction of intense emotion and psychological turmoil. It portrays a skeletal, ghostly figure standing on a bridge against a tumultuous sky, with a landscape of swirling colors and forms. While the painting itself does not explicitly convey the idea that "you can't outrun a memory," it resonates with themes of existential angst, anxiety, and the human experience of overwhelming internal states that can be difficult to escape.

In modern times, similar ideas can be found in psychological literature and self-help books, where the importance of addressing and integrating past experiences into one's current life is frequently discussed. The phrase itself might have gained popularity through its use in songs (see the next essay), books, movies, or even therapeutic contexts, where the struggle to manage and reconcile with one's memories is a common theme.

In the context of psychological health, this phrase underscores the importance of addressing past experiences rather than avoiding them. For patients dealing with trauma, unresolved memories can manifest as anxiety, depression, or PTSD. Therapeutic approaches, such as cognitive-behavioral therapy (CBT), eye movement desensitization and reprocessing (EMDR), or narrative therapy, are often employed to help individuals process and integrate these memories in a healthy way.

For physicians and healthcare providers, understanding that patients may be dealing with persistent and intrusive memories is crucial. It informs a compassionate approach to care, where the focus is not only on physical symptoms but also on the emotional and psychological well-being of the patient. Creating a safe and supportive environment where patients feel comfortable discussing their past can be a significant step towards healing.

Administratively, this concept can influence the development of patient care protocols that prioritize mental health screenings and the integration of mental health services into primary care. It also highlights the need for ongoing education and training for healthcare providers in trauma-informed care practices.

Here are some clinical examples that illustrate the concept "You Can't Outrun a Memory":

Example 1: Post-Traumatic Stress

Patient: A 35-year-old military veteran.

History: The patient served in active combat and witnessed traumatic events. After returning home, he experiences recurring nightmares, flashbacks, and severe anxiety.

Clinical Presentation: The patient avoids places, people, and activities that remind him of his service. Despite moving to a new city and changing jobs, his symptoms persist and interfere with daily functioning.

Intervention: The clinician recommends cognitive-behavioral therapy (CBT) and eye movement desensitization and reprocessing (EMDR) to help process and integrate the traumatic memories. The patient is also started on a selective serotonin reuptake inhibitor (SSRI) to help manage anxiety and depression.

Outcome: Through therapy, the patient learns coping strategies and gradually reduces the intensity of his flashbacks and nightmares. Although the memories do not disappear, he gains better control over his reactions to them.

Example 2: Childhood Abuse

Patient: A 28-year-old woman with a history of childhood physical abuse.

History: The patient experienced physical abuse from a caregiver during her childhood. She now struggles with trust issues, low self-esteem, and chronic depression.

Clinical Presentation: Despite relocating to a different city and cutting ties with her abuser, she continues to experience intrusive memories and emotional distress, particularly in intimate relationships.

Intervention: The clinician uses trauma-focused therapy, such as trauma-focused CBT (TF-CBT), to help the patient work through her past experiences. Group therapy is also suggested to provide support from others with similar experiences.

Outcome: Over time, the patient develops healthier coping mechanisms and begins to form more trusting relationships. The memories of the abuse remain, but they no longer dominate her emotional landscape.

Example 3: Loss and Grief

Patient: A 50-year-old man who lost his spouse unexpectedly.

History: The patient's spouse died suddenly from a heart attack two years ago. Since then, he has struggled with unrelenting grief and depression.

Clinical Presentation: He avoids places and activities that remind him of his spouse. He moved to a new home, hoping that a change of environment would help, but he continues to feel overwhelmed by sadness and loneliness.

Intervention: The clinician recommends grief counseling and possibly joining a support group for people who have lost loved ones. The patient is also evaluated for antidepressant medication to help manage his depressive symptoms.

Outcome: The patient is started on an SSRI antidepressant. Through counseling and support, he learns to express his grief and finds ways to honor his spouse's memory. He begins to re-engage with life and find joy in new activities, though he continues to carry the memory of his spouse with him.

Example 4: Substance Use

Patient: A 40-year-old man with a history of alcohol use disorder.

History: The patient began drinking heavily in his twenties to cope with the stress of a high-pressure job and unresolved childhood trauma.

Clinical Presentation: Although he has been in remission for a year and attends regular AA meetings, he continues to experience intense cravings and guilt associated with his past behavior.

Intervention: The clinician suggests continued participation in a 12-step program and introduces individual therapy sessions that focus on addressing the underlying trauma and developing healthier coping strategies.

Outcome: The patient gains a deeper understanding of the root causes of his addiction and learns to manage his cravings more effectively. While the memories of his past struggles with alcohol remain, they no longer dictate his actions.

These examples illustrate the enduring impact of significant memories and the importance of therapeutic interventions to help patients process and integrate these experiences into their lives in a healthy way.

"You Can't Outrun a Memory" serves as a reminder of the lasting impact of our experiences and the importance of addressing them with empathy and professional support.

36. You Can't Outrun the Truth

The undeniable reality of the coronavirus pandemic became impossible to ignore.

The phrase "you can't outrun the truth" is a maxim like "you can't outrun a memory." Both sayings encapsulate a universal human experience rather than having a well-documented origin or attribution to a specific author. Both phrases convey the idea that certain aspects of our internal or external reality – be it memories or truths – cannot be avoided, no matter how much one might try to escape or deny them.

Both phrases emphasize the idea of inescapability. Whether it's the truth or a memory, these elements will persist despite attempts to ignore, avoid, or flee from them. Additionally, both concepts highlight the psychological struggle of dealing with internal realities. Memories and truths can have significant emotional and mental impacts that need to be addressed rather than avoided. Implicit in both phrases is the suggestion that confronting these realities is necessary for genuine resolution or peace, as avoidance often leads to prolonged distress or unresolved issues.

However, there are differences between the two phrases. "You can't outrun a memory" focuses on personal, often emotional experiences and the persistence of past events in one's mind. In contrast, "You can't outrun the truth" is broader and can apply to both internal and external realities, including facts, realities, or outcomes that exist independently of one's internal experiences. The memory phrase is often used in contexts dealing with trauma, regret, or past experiences, whereas the truth phrase is frequently used in contexts of honesty, accountability, and acceptance of reality, whether personal or public.

For instance, consider a clinical example involving a 55-year-old man with symptoms of a serious illness. Despite experiencing symptoms, he avoids seeking medical advice due to fear of a potential diagnosis.

The clinician emphasizes the importance of confronting the truth about his health to address any issues early and improve outcomes. Eventually, the patient seeks medical evaluation, which leads to early detection and better management of his condition.

Another example involves a 30-year-old woman experiencing anxiety and panic attacks. She avoids acknowledging the underlying stressors in her life, such as a toxic relationship and job dissatisfaction. Through therapy, the clinician helps her recognize and confront the truth about her life circumstances. By facing these truths, she begins to make necessary changes, leading to improved mental health.

"Can't Outrun the Truth" is a song composed in 2021 by The Who legend Pete Townshend and his wife Rachel Fuller. It was sparked by the emotional challenges people faced during the COVID-19 pandemic-induced isolation and the lack of human interaction. Fuller felt that young people, in particular those undergoing cancer treatment, may identify with these feelings of isolation. Townshend perceived, "If you've got a scenario in which somebody in your family or a teenager has got cancer, they're being treated, lockdown hits, and you're not allowed to go and visit them. There's a poignancy to the whole thing about the song."

Indeed, the phrase "you can't outrun the truth" was particularly relevant to the coronavirus pandemic, especially when considering the prevalence of conspiracy theories, science denial, and vaccine refusal that surrounded the virus, leading many to doubt the severity of the pandemic or the benefits of vaccination (refer to essay 12). These unfounded beliefs not only hindered efforts to control the virus but also fostered a climate of distrust and fear. However, as the pandemic progressed, the stark reality of COVID-19's impact became impossible to ignore. The mounting numbers of infections, hospitalizations, and deaths served as a grim reminder that the virus was a real and present danger, unaffected by the whims of misinformation.

Science denial regarding the effectiveness of vaccines and public health measures posed the most significant obstacles. Some individuals refused to wear masks, practice social distancing, or get vaccinated, often citing personal freedoms or skepticism about scientific recommendations. Yet, the data consistently showed that COVID-19 vaccines, like other types of vaccines, were highly effective in preventing severe illness and death, and that public health measures can significantly reduce transmission. The persistence of the virus in communities with low vaccination rates underscored the reality that disregarding scientific evidence has tangible, often dire, consequences.

In the face of vaccine refusal, the adage "you can't outrun the truth" became even more apparent. Vaccines were the critical tool in reducing the spread of COVID-19 and mitigating its impact. However, vaccine hesitancy allowed the virus to continue circulating, leading to new variants and prolonged societal disruption. Ultimately, the truth of the virus's threat and the efficacy of vaccines became undeniable. The longer vaccine refusal persisted, the more evident it became that embracing scientific truth was essential for overcoming the pandemic.

"You can't outrun the truth" can be interpreted in several other meaningful ways in relation to the coronavirus pandemic to reflect aspects of personal responsibility, social inequities, global interconnectedness, long-term consequences, and the importance of trust in leadership. In all scenarios, the underlying message remains clear: facing and accepting the truth is essential for effective response and recovery.

Both phrases – "you can't outrun a memory" and "you can't outrun the truth" – serve as reminders that avoidance is not a viable long-term strategy for dealing with significant internal or external realities, much less the threat of a global pandemic.

37. The "Dainty Maids"

The U.S. Supreme Court "Dobbs" decision has reversed decades of reproductive rights progress that began with the "Dainty Maids."

The term "Dainty Maids" could refer to various subjects depending on the context – ranging from historical groups to fictional characters.

Historically, women in service roles, such as maids or attendants, were referred to as Dainty Maids. They were noted for their refined manners and appearance, women who embodied ideals of delicacy and decorum. In literary works, poetry, and plays from various periods, particularly in the Victorian era, Dainty Maids were often described with particular attention to their elegance and grace. These characters might be depicted as young women of high social standing or those serving in noble households.

"Dainty Maid" has also been used as a brand name for various products over the years. For example, in the mid-20th century, Dainty Maid was a brand of baking products, including cake mixes and other dessert items. These products were marketed to homemakers with an emphasis on creating delicate and delicious treats.

Around this time (1950s), women known as "Dainty Maids" surfaced selling door-to-door feminine hygiene products while covertly distributing contraceptives. This was a significant and somewhat clandestine effort during a time when birth control was a controversial and legally restricted topic: birth control was illegal in the U.S. until 1965 (for married couples) and 1972 (for single people).

In the 1950s, women had limited options for family planning and faced significant challenges if they wanted to control their reproductive health. Diaphragms were the only contraceptives for women. There was a catch, however. Most gynecologists would fit only married or engaged women – no "singles." Many practices saw quite a number of very young (14 or 15-year-old) pregnant girls and sent them to maternity homes, which are back in vogue as a result of the reversal of Roe v Wade in 2022 by the U.S. Supreme Court. The "Dobbs" ruling that has supplanted "Roe" has essentially denied abortion and some forms of contraception in many states.

The "Dainty Maids" played a crucial role in providing access to contraceptives. They worked under the guise of selling feminine hygiene products, which were socially acceptable and did not raise suspicion. This allowed them to enter homes and offer information and products related to birth control (often spermicides) in a discreet manner. The Dainty Maids' work was therefore not just socially risky but also legally perilous.

The legacy of the Dainty Maids is significant. Their efforts led to more widespread acceptance and eventual legalization of contraceptives. Their bravery and commitment to women's health and rights laid the groundwork for future advancements in reproductive health. These women were pioneers, and their actions contributed to the gradual change in societal attitudes towards contraception and women's health culminating in the groundbreaking 1973 "Roe" decision.

We are now witnessing a concerning reversal in the progress made toward women's reproductive rights, spurred by recent legal and ideological shifts. "Dobbs" has played a significant role in setting back five decades of precedent and undermining the Constitution's promise of freedom and equality for women, catalyzing the rise of restrictive reproductive laws and attitudes. More than two years after the fall of "Roe," healthcare providers are still unable to provide standard medical care in states with abortion bans, leading to delays, denials of care, and worsened health outcomes, deepening the existing inequities in the health care system for people of color.

The impact of these changes is notable, affecting not only women's health – teenagers and young women in particular – but also their social and economic well-being. Restricted access to reproductive health services can lead to higher rates of unintended pregnancies, which in turn can perpetuate cycles of poverty and limit women's opportunities for education and employment. The ideological underpinnings of this movement often stem from deeply held beliefs about gender roles and the sanctity of life, which are being translated into policies that prioritize fetal rights over women's rights. As a result, an increasingly robust body of evidence is emerging that clearly illustrates Dobbs is harming reproductive health and freedom as well as fundamentally changing the nature of obstetric care.

The medical community, including doctors and professional organizations, has been vocal in its response to the Dobbs decision and the subsequent legislative changes that restrict access to reproductive health services. The American Medical Association (AMA), for example, has strongly opposed the Dobbs decision, stating that it undermines the patient-physician relationship and interferes with medical practice. The organization emphasizes that decisions about reproductive health should be made by patients in consultation with their physicians, without political interference, and doctors should not be threatened with incarceration for performing medically necessary procedures that run afoul of states' laws.

Similarly, the American College of Obstetricians and Gynecologists (ACOG) has been a staunch advocate for reproductive rights and has condemned the Dobbs decision. ACOG argues that access to safe and legal abortion is a critical component of comprehensive healthcare and that restrictions on abortion services compromise the health and safety of women. The American Academy of Family Physicians (AAFP) has also expressed concern about the impact of restrictive abortion laws on the ability of family physicians to provide comprehensive care. The organization supports access to the full spectrum of reproductive health services, including abortion, and opposes legislation that interferes with the patient-physician relationship.

The National Medical Association (NMA), representing African American physicians, has highlighted the disproportionate impact of restrictive reproductive laws on marginalized communities. The organization advocates for equitable access to reproductive healthcare and opposes policies that exacerbate health disparities. Many individual physicians have taken to public forums, including social media, op-eds, and professional conferences, to express their opposition to the Dobbs decision. They often share personal stories and clinical experiences to illustrate the negative consequences of restricted access to reproductive health services.

In response to these challenges, some medical schools and residency programs are adjusting their curricula to ensure that future physicians are trained in providing comprehensive reproductive healthcare, including abortion services, despite the legal challenges. Additionally, medical organizations are collaborating with legal, advocacy, and human rights groups to challenge restrictive laws and to provide support for patients seeking reproductive healthcare. These collaborations aim to safeguard access to care and to protect physicians who provide these services from legal repercussions.

It is vital to recognize the historical context and the struggles that led to the advancements in reproductive rights given that they have come under attack again. The efforts of past advocates like the Dainty Maids highlight the importance of continued advocacy and education to protect and advance women's health and autonomy. The current climate calls for renewed vigilance and activism to safeguard the hard-won gains in reproductive rights and to ensure that future generations do not face the same barriers.

38. The Persistent Shadows of Barbarism in Medicine

Stark reminders of past misadventures are cautionary tales for the future.

Barbarism in medicine is characterized by practices that are cruel, inhumane, or primitive by modern standards. These practices have marred the history of medical science from antiquity through modern times, often shaped by a lack of understanding of human physiology, superstition, and the prevailing cultural and religious beliefs of the era. While many of these practices were intended to heal, they frequently resulted in harm, revealing the dark side of the history of medicine. This darkness has cast shadows on the evolution of medical knowledge, highlighting the trial-and-error nature of early treatments and the often-dire consequences for patients. These shadows unfortunately persist today.

Ancient Times

In ancient times, medical practices were deeply intertwined with religion and mysticism. The Egyptians, for example, believed that disease was caused by evil spirits or the wrath of the gods. As a result, treatments often involved rituals and offerings to appease these supernatural forces. One particularly barbaric practice was trepanation, the drilling or scraping of a hole into the skull of a living person. This procedure, which dates back thousands of years, was believed to release evil spirits or relieve pressure on the brain. However, without anesthesia or a proper understanding of antisepsis, this procedure was incredibly painful and often fatal.

The Greeks and Romans, though more advanced in their medical understanding, also engaged in practices that would be considered barbaric by today's standards. Hippocrates advocated for the use of bloodletting to balance the body's humors – blood, phlegm, black bile, and yellow bile. This practice was based on the belief that illness was caused by an imbalance of these humors. Bloodletting, often performed using leeches or by cutting a vein, persisted for centuries despite its unproven efficacy and the dangers of excessive blood loss.

Middle Ages, Renaissance, and Enlightenment

During the Middle Ages, the practice of medicine in Europe became even more intertwined with religious dogma. The Church exerted significant control over medical practices, and many treatments were based on religious beliefs rather than scientific evidence. For example, exorcisms were commonly performed to cure mental illness, which was often believed to be caused by demonic possession. The use of relics, prayers, and pilgrimages as cures for physical ailments was also widespread. These practices, though rooted in faith, often led to the suffering and death of patients who might have survived with proper medical attention.

The period's limited medical knowledge and slow scientific progress contributed to the role of barbers in medical practices, which in turn gave rise to the term "barbarism." Barbers played a critical role in early medical procedures, especially those that were somewhat rudimentary and often brutal by modern standards.

In medieval Europe, barbers were not just responsible for cutting hair and grooming beards like traditional barbers do today. They also performed surgery, known as "barber-surgeons." These individuals provided a range of services, including bloodletting, tooth extraction, lancing abscesses, and even amputations.

Barber-surgeons operated without the benefits of modern anesthesia, antiseptics, or a deep understanding of human anatomy, which often made their procedures painful and dangerous. The barber-surgeon was a common figure because formal medical practitioners, who were often clergy or scholars, did not typically engage in hands-on medical treatment. Instead, they focused on diagnosis and theoretical aspects of medicine, leaving the practical and often messy work to barber-surgeons.

Surgery was not considered a formal part of medicine during Medieval times. As such, barber-surgeons were typically trained through apprenticeships and seen as more akin to craftsmen than learned scholars. They were actually referred to as “Mister,” a term used for skilled tradesmen, rather than addressed as “doctor.” (Today, in the UK and some other countries, the distinction between “mister” and “doctor” persists as a historical tradition.)

The iconic red and white barber pole is believed to have originated from the dual role of barber-surgeons. The red stripe symbolizes blood, while the white represents the bandages used in bloodletting. The pole itself may have represented the staff that patients held onto during bloodletting to encourage blood flow.

Although the Renaissance and Enlightenment periods brought advancements in medical knowledge and technique, barbaric practices remained prevalent. The anatomical studies of Andreas Vesalius (1514-1564) and the surgical innovations of Ambroise Paré (1510-1590) marked significant progress, albeit experimental and still performed without anesthesia or only crude forms of anesthesia – alcohol, opium, cold, compression and tourniquets – until the advent of anesthesia with ether centuries later (in 1846). Prior to the 19th century, surgeons eager to explore new techniques operated on patients who were fully conscious, leading to excruciating pain and high mortality rates.

The 19th Century

The rise of anatomy as a scientific discipline unfortunately had some unintended consequences – namely, the unscrupulous practice of grave robbing. Bodies were obtained without consent from loved ones and often dissected in public, with little regard for the dignity of the deceased. In the U.S., the remains of Native Americans were frequently taken from their burial sites and used for scientific study and public display. The act of exhuming and stealing from graves is widely considered unethical, illegal, and culturally insensitive. It is often viewed as a form of barbarism.

A notorious example occurred in 1862. Under orders from President Abraham Lincoln, 38 Native American men of the Santee Dakota people were hanged in the largest mass execution in U.S. history. William W. Mayo, MD, founder of the Mayo Clinic, led a team of doctors who dug up the sacred graves of the executed men and hauled them away for use as medical cadavers. Mayo was given the body of "Cut Nose" (Marpiya te najin, or He Who Stands in the Clouds), the Dakota leader, which he brought to his office, dissected, melted away the flesh, and made a skeleton that he could study and allow his children to play with. (In 2018, Gary RedOwl, a descendent of Marpiya te najin, received a written apology from the Mayo Clinic.)

Many other instances of egregious and barbaric defaming and disrespecting of Native Americans led to a greater awareness and eventual legal changes regarding the treatment of their remains. The Native American Graves Protection and Repatriation Act (NAGPRA) was enacted in 1990 to address these issues, requiring institutions to return human remains and cultural items to their respective tribes and descendants. Yet, institutions have been extremely slow to comply with the law. Many of the nation's top museums and universities have thousands of unauthorized human remains in their collections while tribes still wait for their return.

The 20th and 21st Centuries

Psychiatric Treatment

Few areas in the annals of medicine exhibit more horrific acts of barbarism than the treatment of the mentally ill. The history of psychiatry is dotted with examples of treatments that were believed to have extremely high potential for treating and curing mental illness yet it has almost never been the case that those original expectations were fulfilled.

For example, although the concept of "asylum" for mentally ill patients was rooted in humanitarian considerations, individuals were often subjected to inhumane conditions where they were chained, beaten, and neglected. Treatments such as the "swinging chair" were designed to induce vomiting through intolerable vertigo that supposedly balanced the humors. These swings and cold-water treatments were rapidly adopted in the 1800s across Europe and North America and ended after public and professional opinion turned against such violent methods of therapy – only to favor an even more barbaric treatment: lobotomy

Popularized in the early 20th century as a treatment for various mental illnesses, lobotomy involved severing connections in the brain's prefrontal cortex. This procedure, often performed without the patient's consent or under dubious conditions, resulted in severe cognitive and emotional impairments, sometimes leaving patients in a vegetative state (think: "Mac" [Jack Nicholson] in *One Flew Over the Cuckoo's Nest*).

The tragic case of Rosemary Kennedy, the oldest sister of President John F. Kennedy, who was left incapacitated after a lobotomy (for treatment of an intellectual and disability disorder), highlights the devastating consequences of this practice. Despite initial acclaim, lobotomy is now widely condemned as a barbaric and unethical treatment, reflecting the dangers of medical interventions conducted without sufficient understanding or regard for patient welfare.

The use of electroconvulsive therapy (ECT) without anesthesia or proper safeguards is another example of how psychiatric patients were treated as less than human. Physical injuries, such as fractured bones (particularly vertebrae), dislocated joints, and broken teeth often resulted. The absence of anesthesia meant that patients were fully conscious and aware of the procedure, which could cause substantial psychological distress and trauma.

The debate over the use of solitary confinement in prisons and "seclusion" in psychiatric hospitals raises serious ethical concerns. While short-term seclusion (hours) is often used with mechanical restraints and is intended to protect patients and staff, prolonged isolation can exacerbate mental health issues and cause significant psychological harm. The United Nations has recognized solitary confinement for more than 15 days as a form of torture. This modern-day example of barbarism highlights the need for humane treatment approaches that prioritize patient well-being and recovery. It also calls attention to the need for drastic reform of the prison system, where nearly half of inmates have a diagnosable mental disorder.

The egregious use of seclusion occurs in the form of patient entrapment. The *New York Times* described how a leading chain of for-profit psychiatric hospitals trapped patients and held them against their will to maximize insurance payouts. Investigators determined that detaining patients was not medically necessary and violated the law, requiring judges to intervene for their release. When questioned, patients said they had been kept at the hospitals "with no excuses or valid reason." None of them appeared to have met the legal standard for involuntary commitment, i.e., imminent danger to self or others. Many patients have gone on record stating that forced, involuntary stays have permanently psychologically scarred them.

Eugenics

The eugenics movement of the 20th century was perhaps one of the most infamous examples of barbarism in medical practice. Eugenics, the belief in improving the genetic quality of the human population, led to the forced sterilization of thousands of individuals deemed "unfit" to reproduce – people with disabilities, indigenous women, and women of color – justified by pseudoscientific beliefs about genetic purity and social betterment.

In the U.S., the Supreme Court case Buck v. Bell (1927) upheld the constitutionality of forced sterilization, leading to the sterilization of over 60,000 people in subsequent decades. Similar practices were adopted in other countries, including Nazi Germany, where the eugenics movement culminated in the horrific medical experiments conducted in concentration camps during World War II (refer to essay 13).

The Tuskegee "Experiment"

Another glaring example of barbarism in medicine is the Tuskegee Syphilis Study, discussed in essay 12. The experiment was conducted between 1932 and 1972 by the U.S. Public Health Service. In this study, hundreds of African American men with syphilis were deliberately left untreated to observe the natural progression of the disease. The men were misled about their condition and denied access to effective treatments, even after penicillin became widely available.

The study, which caused immense suffering and death, is a profound violation of ethical standards and a stark example of racial discrimination in medical research. The Tuskegee Syphilis Study underscores the critical need for informed consent, transparency, and respect for all patients, regardless of their background. It also serves as a stark reminder of how medical research can be perverted when it loses sight of the humanity of its subjects.

The "Lysol" Douche

The explicit advertising and marketing of the "Lysol" douche to women in the early to mid-20th century is another disturbing example of barbarism in medicine. Marketed as a feminine hygiene product and even as a contraceptive, douche ads were seen in popular women's magazines such as *Cosmopolitan* and *McCalls* from the 1920s through the 1950s. These douche solutions carried such names as Lysol, Sterizol, and Zonite. The so-called disinfectants destroyed the normal bacteria in the vagina, ironically creating the conditions for disease rather than eliminating them.

Lysol douches in particular contained harmful chemicals that posed serious health risks, including vaginal irritation, burns, infections – and in rare instances, death. The aggressive marketing campaigns exploited societal pressures on women to maintain certain standards of cleanliness and sexual purity, often without regard for their health and well-being. For example, newspaper ad executives notoriously faulted women for bad vaginal hygiene, which they claimed led to bad odors and bad marriages, condoning cheating husbands as if women were to blame for their husbands' infidelity.

Lysol's advertising campaign made it the best-selling method of contraception during the Great Depression, yet hundreds of people died from exposure to it. (As early as 1911, doctors had recorded 193 Lysol poisonings and five deaths from uterine irrigation.) This practice highlights the dangers of commercial interests overriding medical ethics and the importance of protecting consumers from harmful medical products.

Other Vulnerable Populations

In modern times, while explicit barbarism is less prevalent, subtler forms still exist. Reports of coerced sterilization continue to surface, such as the allegations of forced hysterectomies in U.S. immigration detention centers and the exploitation of vulnerable populations in clinical trials (refer to essay 11). In some cases, research participants are not fully informed about the risks involved or are coerced into participating due to economic pressures. The lack of proper ethical oversight in these situations can lead to exploitation and harm, echoing the barbaric practices of the past and underscoring the need for robust protections against medical abuses.

The use of untested and experimental treatments without proper oversight or patient consent was paramount in the infamous case of Paolo Macchiarini, MD, a thoracic surgeon and researcher who gained international fame for his work in regenerative medicine. Macchiarini implanted synthetic ("bioartificial") windpipes into patients. The procedure involved replacing a damaged trachea with a plastic replica that had been soaked in the patient's stem cells. However, the surgery was performed without adequate evidence of safety or efficacy, and resulted in severe complications and multiple patient deaths. Dr. Macchiarini's surgical misadventures and his personal exploits, as discussed in the next essay, were the subject of Peacock's "Dr. Death" season 2 and Netflix's "Bad Surgeon: Love Under the Knife."

Macchiarini was found to have falsified data in his research publications, exaggerating the effectiveness of his procedures while downplaying or outright ignoring the adverse reactions experienced by his patients. In 2022, he was found criminally liable by a Swedish court for causing felony bodily injury to a Turkish woman he had fitted with one of the windpipes at Karolinska University Hospital in Stockholm in 2012. The patient died in 2017 after a lung-trachea transplant at Temple University Hospital in Philadelphia failed to save her life. This case highlights the dangers of prioritizing scientific ambition over patient safety and the critical importance of rigorous ethical standards in medical research.

The Future

Despite these grim aspects, the persistent quest for better understanding and improved therapeutic methods has led to significant medical advancements, laying the foundation for the evidence-based practices that define modern practice today. Still, when acts of medical barbarism are viewed through a historical lens, it begs the question: "What procedures, surgeries, treatments, etc., rendered today might be similarly perceived as 'barbaric' in the future?"

One area that might be scrutinized is the use of certain invasive surgeries. As discussed above, procedures such as lobotomies, once considered cutting-edge treatments for mental illness, are now viewed as inhumane. Similarly, current surgical interventions that involve significant risks and long recovery periods might one day be seen as unnecessarily brutal, especially as minimally invasive techniques and regenerative medicine advance.

Another potential area of future critique could be the over-prescription of medications. The widespread use of powerful psychotropic drugs to manage mental health conditions, despite their efficacy, might be questioned due to their serious side effects. Future generations might view the reliance on these medications as a crude approach, especially if new, more refined medications are developed, or holistic and less pharmacologically reliant treatments become available.

The treatment of chronic pain is also a candidate for future scrutiny. The opioid crisis has already highlighted the dangers of overprescribing painkillers. Future medical professionals might look back on the liberal use of opioids and other addictive substances as a form of medical barbarism, especially if more effective and safer pain management techniques are developed or potent analgesics are introduced without the risk of addiction.

Additionally, the handling of end-of-life care might come under fire. Current practices that prolong life at the expense of quality of life, often involving aggressive treatments with little hope of recovery, might be viewed as inhumane. Advances in palliative care and a better understanding of the importance of quality of life could shift perspectives on what constitutes compassionate care.

Conclusion

Fortunately, some of the past medical wrongs have been righted. With the introduction of anesthesia, muscle relaxants, and proper monitoring, the safety and efficacy of ECT have significantly improved. These advancements have made ECT a life-saving treatment option for severely depressed patients, now accompanied by a much lower risk profile. Likewise, several neurological alternatives to lobotomy are considered acceptable and more effective: deep brain stimulation, transcranial magnetic stimulation, and vagus nerve stimulation.

Barbarism in medicine, whether historical or contemporary, serves as a powerful reminder of the ethical responsibilities inherent in the medical profession. As medical knowledge and technology continue to evolve, practices that are considered standard today might be re-evaluated and deemed barbaric by future standards. This ongoing reassessment underscores the need to uphold the highest ethical standards, prioritize patient welfare, and remain vigilant against practices that dehumanize or harm individuals. Only through a steadfast commitment to ethical principles can the medical community ensure that the mistakes of the past are not repeated and that all patients are treated with dignity and respect.

39. The Dark Psychology of Con-Men in White Coats

Unimaginable tales of deception were perpetrated by physicians.

As I discussed in the previous essay, Paolo Macchiarini, MD, was once a celebrated surgeon who fell from grace due to his unethical practices and personal deceit, destroying the lives of patients and families in his wake.

Farid Fata, MD, is a Lebanese-born Detroit area hematologist-oncologist who was sentenced in 2015 to serve 45 years in prison for his role in a health care fraud scheme that included administering medically unnecessary infusions or injections to 553 individual patients and submitting to Medicare and private insurance companies approximately $34 million in fraudulent claims. He caused grievous emotional and physical harm to patients by falsely diagnosing them with cancer and providing unnecessary chemotherapy.

Michael Swango, MD, is a physician who became a serial killer. He poisoned patients and colleagues, and manipulated his way through multiple medical institutions, leaving a trail of mysterious patient deaths, possibly as many as 60. His charm and ability to deceive colleagues and law enforcement authorities allowed him to evade detection for 20 years while he continued his killing spree. Swango was sentenced in 2000 to three consecutive life terms without the possibility of parole.

All of these doctors exploited their positions of power, relying on the assumption that physicians are inherently trustworthy and competent. They illustrate that the allure of power and recognition can sometimes lead individuals down a very dark path, and they are a stark reminder that even medicine is not immune to the actions of swindlers and con-men.

Throughout history, there have been other medical professionals involved in fraudulent activities, typically motivated by ambition, narcissism, and a quest for fame or financial gain. However, it seems that none have crafted stories as sensational as Macchiarini. In the words of Meredith Vieira: "He's the doctor who does the seemingly impossible, going where no other has yet dared."

Just ask Benita Alexander, an Emmy award-winning journalist and producer who was responsible for the documentary *A Leap of Faith*, hosted by Vieira and aired on NBC on June 1, 2016. While filming was occurring in 2013, Alexander fell in love with Macchiarini, the subject of the documentary. Apart from her breach of journalistic ethics, Alexander was swept into a marriage proposal and lavish wedding plans that Macchiarini said would be officiated by Pope Francis and include Elton John and John Legend for entertainment. Andrea Bocelli was to serenade the couple, and attendees would include the Obamas, the Clintons, and other dignitaries and celebrities

The reckoning occurred when Alexander learned that Macchiarini's peripatetic studies and distinguished medical pedigree were half-baked (think: George Santos). She discovered with the help of a private investigator that virtually every detail Macchiarini provided about the wedding was false. Additionally, he was living with a woman and two children in Barcelona, and it was not entirely certain whether Macchiarini had actually obtained a legal divorce from his first wife.

Macchiarini's Munchausen life was outlined in *Vanity Fair* (February 2016 issue). Ronald Schouten, MD, JD, Director of the Law & Psychiatry Service and the MGH/Harvard Forensic Psychiatry Fellowship, and an Associate Professor of Psychiatry at Harvard Medical School was interviewed for the article and quoted as saying, "Macchiarini is the extreme form of a con man. He's clearly bright and has accomplishments, but he can't contain himself. There's a void in his personality that he seems to want to fill by conning more and more people…This guy is *really* good."

The psychology of con-men in medicine often involves complex personality traits and psychological disorders. Many con-men exhibit characteristics of narcissistic personality disorder, which includes an inflated sense of self-importance, a need for excessive admiration, and a lack of empathy for others. These traits can drive individuals to manipulate and deceive people to maintain their self-image and achieve their goals. In the context of medicine, this can manifest as falsifying research, performing unnecessary procedures, or lying about qualifications and achievements.

The relationship between con-men and medicine is particularly troubling because it undermines the trust that is fundamental to the doctor-patient relationship. Medicine is a field that requires a high degree of trust, both from patients who rely on their doctors for life-saving treatments and from the broader community that expects medical professionals to adhere to ethical standards. When a con-man infiltrates this field, the consequences can be devastating, leading not only to the erosion of public trust and damage to the reputation of the medical profession and institutions but also loss of life and deep psychological trauma for victims and their families.

Con-men in medicine are often able to exploit the inherent vulnerabilities in the healthcare system, such as the complexity of medical knowledge and the emotional and financial stakes involved in healthcare decisions. They may use their charm and intelligence to gain the confidence of colleagues and patients, and they can be remarkably adept at manipulating systems to their advantage. This makes it all the more important for medical institutions to have robust oversight mechanisms and for the medical community to remain vigilant against unethical and unprofessional behavior or substandard practice.

For example, during Swango's residency at Ohio State University (OSU), several patients under his care experienced unexplained complications and deaths. Despite suspicions and internal investigations, the university did not initially take decisive action, allowing Swango to complete his internship (but he was not invited back for a neurosurgery residency). His eventual conviction led to recriminations at OSU. A scathing review by James Meeks, who was the dean of OSU's law school at the time, concluded that the hospital should have called in the police, and also revealed several flagrant shortcomings in its initial investigation, calling it "far too superficial." Meeks' report served as a wake-up call for the medical community, emphasizing the need for mechanisms to promptly address potential criminal activities within healthcare settings.

Many scholars since then have recognized that the field of medicine, with its hierarchical structures and reverence for authority, can provide fertile ground for con-men. The culture of deference to senior physicians and the assumption of competence based on credentials can allow con-men to thrive. Their presence in the profession serves as a cautionary tale about the dangers of unchecked power and the importance of monitoring for imbalances. While medical con-men are outliers, their impact is overwhelming, underscoring the need for systems of accountability and the cultivation of a medical culture that prioritizes ethics and competence over ego and greed.

40. I Trusted Con-"Men in Black," but Thankfully Not with My Health

If health care were modeled after the automotive industry, what would be the consequences?

I traded my beloved 2017 Mercedes Benz for a 2025 Kia Sorrento hybrid. I thought I should reduce my carbon footprint and drive a hybrid car (e-vehicles have yet to win me over). The dealership was completely focused on making the sale, and they left me in the dust afterwards. I shouldn't have expected anything more from an automotive chain named after a famous race car driver, one who was also famous for leaving his competitors in the dust. The dealership's namesake may have been a world-class race car driver, but he was a second-rate role model for a business, especially in health care.

I noticed that during the buying process, the salespeople took their marching orders from higher-ups situated behind an opaque glass-protected fortress situated on the side of the showroom. No one stationed inside came out to greet me. Instead, the salespeople would go into the room and shortly emerge like zombies with numbers scribbled on a piece of paper. They dressed in sleek all-back apparel.

I wasn't satisfied with the initial offer, so I asked my salesperson if I could visit his High Holiness inside the fortress. I was able to negotiate a better deal directly with the sales manager than I was with my messenger salesperson – and without his back-and-forth trips to the fortress.

I purchased my new car on a Sunday. I picked it up the next day at 3 pm. The pinstripe, which was paid and promised, was missing. The salesperson allotted only 10 minutes to go over the complicated electronic settings, confessing that some of the electronics were even "too new" for him. My salesperson told me to schedule a time to come back to have the pinstripe applied. He also promise all-weather floormats in return for a 10-star review of his services. He said, "Call me when you receive the satisfaction survey from Kia in your email so we can do it together. I need all 10s and nothing less."

During subsequent attempts to reach him by phone I was always told he was with a "guest" and would call me back. It took 2 weeks to connect with him. I discovered that my Mercedes Benz was listed for sale on their website for $32,600, although I was given only $25,000 as a trade-in allowance – the dealer's "best" price, according to the sales manager.

While this scenario, unfortunately, is not uncommon in the automotive industry, imagining such practices in healthcare offers a stark contrast and raises important considerations about the values and ethics across different sectors. Drawing a parallel helps us understand how detrimental such an approach could be if applied to healthcare operations.

First, the dealership's decision-making process was shrouded in secrecy. If healthcare providers operated similarly, taking orders from unseen managers without explaining treatment plans to patients, it would lead to a lack of trust and understanding about one's health care. This impersonal approach could severely undermine the patient-provider relationship, which is fundamental to effective health care.

Second, the lack of personal interaction, where there were no overtures from management and no manager available to speak to me directly unless I requested it, would be equally problematic in health care. It's like never meeting the attending physician in charge of the healthcare team and decision making. If doctors and healthcare providers never personally engaged with their patients, it would result in a cold and impersonal experience, potentially negatively impacting patient outcomes. Personal interaction and communication are critical components of patient care, fostering trust and ensuring that patients feel valued and understood.

Third, the pressure for a perfect review – and an offer of all-weather floor mats in exchange – would be unethical if applied in health care. Imagine healthcare practitioners pressuring patients to give perfect satisfaction scores in exchange for better treatment or faster service. This could lead to compromised care quality and unscrupulous practices, as providers might prioritize ratings over genuine patient care.

Fourth, my experience at the car dealer involved incomplete service and poor follow-up, e.g., the missing pinstripe and the salesperson's inadequate guidance on electronic settings. If patients left the hospital without all prescribed treatments or follow-up care, it could lead to deteriorating health conditions and potentially severe consequences. Discharge instructions coupled with effective follow-up and comprehensive care are essential to ensure patient compliance and positive health outcomes (refer to essay 18).

Financial transparency is a fifth critical issue highlighted by my experience. Discovering that my trade-in was significantly undervalued is frustrating, and in a healthcare context, a lack of transparency in billing and treatment costs could lead to patients being overcharged or not fully aware of their financial obligations. No wonder there was bipartisan agreement to pass the "No Surprises Act" in 2022. It protects patients from unexpected out-of-network medical bills and "sticker shock" associated with emergency department treatment. Yet, many patients are *still* unaware of what they're going to be paying, due to the complicated puzzle of insurance.

Sixth, the "Men in Black" routine would never work in health care. While many hospitals promulgate and enforce dress codes, they tend not to be as draconian as the ones I've witnessed at car dealerships and other service-oriented establishments. Doctors' suits and ties are hospital décor of the past. Besides, ties carry germs and spread infection!

Unlike car sales, where a dissatisfied customer can eventually sell or trade in a car, people have only one body, and it must be maintained for life. Poor or inadequate health care, like a run-down car, can result in long-term breakdowns with life-threatening consequences. My experience highlights the importance of upholding high ethical principles, transparency, and personal interaction in any industry. Applying the practices of a car dealer to health care would be unacceptable and potentially dangerous. Industries should learn from one another and implement best practices to consistently prioritize and earn customer (or patient) satisfaction and trust.

41. The Diligent Patient

John Donne's perspective of healthcare diligence extrapolates to the ideal doctor-patient relationship.

John Donne's quote, "I observe the physician with the same diligence as he the disease," reflects a keen awareness and scrutiny of the physician's methods and actions. Donne (1572-1631), a metaphysical poet and preacher, often explored themes of life, death, and the human condition in his work. In this statement, he implies that just as a physician meticulously studies a disease to diagnose and treat it, Donne, as a patient or an observer, equally scrutinizes the physician's competence, approach, and behavior.

This observation can be interpreted in several ways. Donne might be expressing a cautious trust in the physician's ability, suggesting that patients should be vigilant and well-informed about their treatment and the person administering it. There's a sense of mutual respect and diligence in the relationship between the patient and the physician. Just as the physician is diligent in their duty to heal, the patient is diligent in ensuring they receive proper care.

Donne could also be highlighting the fallibility of physicians, reminding us that they are human and capable of mistakes. Therefore, it is wise for patients to be observant and engaged in their own care. The quote underscores the importance of an active, informed, and observant role for patients in their healthcare, mirroring the dedication and diligence expected from their physicians.

Extrapolating on the Diligent Patient

A long time ago I was asked by a medical student to pontificate on John Donne's quote. I delved deeper into the philosophical and practical implications of his perspective, extending its relevance beyond immediate clinical interactions to broader themes in healthcare and society. I explained to the student that I viewed Donne's position as fundamental to the dynamics of trust, responsibility, and diligence in the patient-physician relationship. This observation is not merely about ensuring competent medical care but also about fostering a deeper understanding of the human condition and the shared journey between patient and healer.

Extrapolating from Donne's perspective, we can explore the idea that diligence in healthcare extends to the systemic and societal levels. For instance, the diligence of patients and physicians can influence healthcare policies, advocate for better healthcare systems, and promote public health initiatives. In this broader context, patients who are diligent and informed can drive changes that improve healthcare accessibility, affordability, and quality for entire communities.

Moreover, Donne's emphasis on observation and diligence can be seen as a call for greater empathy and compassion in health care. Physicians, in their diligent observation of diseases, must also be attuned to the emotional and psychological needs of their patients. This holistic approach to health care, which considers both the physical and mental well-being of patients, aligns with contemporary movements towards integrative and patient-centered care.

On a more philosophical level, Donne's quote can be interpreted as a reflection on the nature of knowledge and the pursuit of understanding. Just as physicians diligently study diseases to uncover their mysteries and find cures, patients, too, must strive to understand their own bodies and health conditions. This mutual pursuit of knowledge fosters a deeper connection between patient and physician, grounded in respect and shared goals.

In the time that has passed since the student asked me to discuss Donne's quote, artificial intelligence and medical technologies have evolved. Donne's call for diligence takes on new dimensions in this light. Both patients and physicians must navigate the complexities of digital health, ensuring that technological advancements enhance rather than hinder the human aspects of care. This requires continuous learning, ethical considerations, and a commitment to preserving the core values of medicine.

Diligent Patient Scenario

From a clinical perspective, a diligent patient is characterized by their consistent and thorough approach to managing their health. This patient meticulously follows prescribed treatments, attends all scheduled appointments, and adheres strictly to medical advice. They maintain detailed records of their symptoms, medications, and any relevant health information, ensuring they are well-prepared for each visit with the doctor. Diligence in healthcare often translates to a high level of compliance with medical recommendations and a structured, methodical approach to health maintenance.

Consider Mr. Thompson, a 60-year-old man with type 2 diabetes. He visits his primary care physician, Sheila Jackson, DO, for his quarterly check-up. Mr. Thompson has been managing his diabetes for the past five years and has consistently adhered to his treatment plan. He arrives at the appointment with a well-organized folder containing his blood sugar logs, a list of medications, and recent lab results, which he has obtained from his patient portal.

During the office visit, Mr. Thompson reviews his blood sugar readings with Dr. Jackson and discusses any minor fluctuations he has noticed. He faithfully follows his prescribed diet and exercise regimen, regularly attends diabetes education classes, and takes his medications as directed. Mr. Thompson also brings up any new symptoms or concerns he has experienced since his last visit, such as occasional tingling in his feet, which he suspects may be related to diabetic neuropathy.

Dr. Jackson appreciates Mr. Thompson's thoroughness and attention to detail. They discuss potential adjustments to his treatment plan, including a slight modification in medication dosage and recommendations for managing neuropathy symptoms. Mr. Thompson takes detailed notes during the consultation and leaves with a clear understanding of the next steps in his care. His diligence ensures that his diabetes remains well-controlled and that any emerging issues are promptly addressed.

Diligent Physician Scenario

Dr. Jackson exemplifies diligence in her approach to managing Mr. Thompson's type 2 diabetes during their quarterly check-up. Before the appointment, Dr. Jackson thoroughly reviews Mr. Thompson's medical history, recent lab results, and notes from previous visits to ensure she is fully informed about his current health status and ongoing treatment plan.

During the visit, Dr. Jackson listens attentively as Mr. Thompson reviews his meticulously kept blood sugar logs, list of medications, and any new symptoms, such as the occasional tingling in his feet. Dr. Jackson appreciates Mr. Thompson's diligence and ensures that their discussion is comprehensive. She asks targeted questions to gain a deeper understanding of Mr. Thompson's daily routine, dietary habits, and any challenges he may be facing in managing his diabetes.

Dr. Jackson employs an ambient AI scribe to summarize the clinical encounter (refer to essay 8), integrating into the electronic health record any changes in Mr. Thompson's condition and the adjustments made to his treatment plan. She provides clear and specific recommendations, including a slight modification in medication dosage and strategies for managing neuropathy symptoms. Additionally, Dr. Jackson schedules a follow-up appointment to monitor Mr. Thompson's progress and encourages him to reach out with any concerns in the interim.

By maintaining thorough and organized patient records, staying updated on the latest diabetes management guidelines, and fostering a collaborative relationship with Mr. Thompson, Dr. Jackson ensures that her patient receives the highest standard of care. Her diligence not only helps in effectively managing Mr. Thompson's diabetes but also strengthens the trust and communication essential for successful long-term health outcomes.

In conclusion, extrapolating on John Donne's quote reveals a multifaceted understanding of healthcare diligence. It underscores the importance of mutual vigilance and responsibility between patients and physicians, while also highlighting broader implications for healthcare systems, empathy, knowledge, and technological integration. Donne's timeless wisdom continues to inspire a thoughtful and comprehensive approach to health and healing in the modern world.

42. Reconnecting with Mentors After the Passage of Time

The ebb and flow of relationships produces currents of wisdom passed down through generations.

Reconnecting with former mentors can be both a nostalgic and enlightening experience, often offering insights into how our past influences have shaped our present. Recently, I decided to reach out to three physicians who played pivotal roles early in my career. Now retired and in their 80s, each left an indelible mark on my professional identity. To rekindle our connection, I sent them an essay (#13 in this book) about the importance of revoking reverence for unethical physicians, a topic that I believed would resonate with their experiences and values.

At the prospect of reestablishing ties, I couldn't help but think of Al Stewart's 1978 hit song "Time Passages," which describes the singer planning a trip home in late December, filled with nostalgic memories of the past. The familiar line "Buy me a ticket on the last train home tonight" reverberated deeply with me, symbolizing my own efforts to revisit and reconnect with these influential figures. Given our shared history and the gravity of the subject matter, I anticipated a thoughtful and engaging dialogue. However, the responses I received were unexpectedly brief and somewhat detached.

Doctor A, an infectious disease specialist, acknowledged the essay with a succinct, "Thanks Arthur. This is an important issue, one that is sometimes hard to navigate. Be well." His response, though polite, lacked the depth of engagement I had hoped for, leaving me wondering about his current perspective and level of interest.

Doctor B, a fellow psychiatrist, offered a similarly brief reply: "Thanks, Art. Well done. Hope that all is good with you and yours.

[Sent from my iPhone]." The casual tone and the note about his device suggested a hurried response, perhaps indicative of a busy or distracted moment. This brevity felt particularly surprising given our shared specialty and intimate patient discussions during my residency.

Doctor C, a medical ethicist, provided the most detailed response, yet it too was marked by a sense of finality: "Dear Art. Thank you for sending this article. It's good to see your continued activism in ethics. I hope all is well with you and your family. I'm fully retired at this point. We sold our home of 50 years and are living in a 2 BR condo. With warm regards." His note, while kind and personal, also conveyed a significant life transition and a possible retreat from professional discourse.

These responses, though courteous, revealed a surprising lack of enthusiasm for rekindling our relationship. This isn't necessarily a negative development; rather, it reflects the natural progression of life and the evolution of personal and professional roles. Our mentors, who once guided us with vigor and insight, may now be navigating different paths, where professional engagement takes a backseat to personal fulfillment and tranquility. While their terse responses initially felt like a missed opportunity for deeper connection, they also served as a valuable lesson in respecting the natural ebb and flow of relationships and the diverse ways in which our mentors choose to engage with their past protégés.

As a practicing psychiatrist, I have always valued the mentor-mentee relationship and the mutual enrichment it brings. My mentors were once vibrant, highly engaged physicians who dedicated their lives to the practice of medicine and the education of future physicians. Their enthusiasm and commitment were contagious, inspiring me and many others to pursue excellence in our fields.

However, as I reconnected with them, I noticed a palpable shift in their demeanor. Their responses, while polite, lacked the warmth and depth I had once experienced. This change, I realized, is not merely a reflection of time passed but also indicative of the natural process of disengagement from the medical profession that comes with aging, retirement, and the health challenges that often accompany these stages of life.

Retirement marks a significant transition in a physician's life. It is a time to step back from the demands of clinical practice, to rest, and to reflect on a career well-lived. For many, it is also a period of adjustment, as they navigate the loss of a professional identity that defined them for decades. The detachment I sensed in my mentors' replies may well be a manifestation of this transition. Having devoted their lives to the service of others, they are now in a phase where they are gradually letting go of their professional ties and embracing a new chapter, perhaps focused on themselves and their families.

The brevity of their responses may also reflect a desire to distance themselves from the emotional and cognitive demands of their former roles. After years of intense intellectual engagement and emotional investment in their patients and students, it is natural for retired physicians to seek a simpler, more tranquil existence. This shift is a healthy and necessary part of aging, allowing them to preserve their well-being and enjoy the fruits of their labor.

Adding to this process are the medical issues that aging brings. For example, I know that Doctor C's wife suffered a stroke several years ago, which was a significant factor in their decision to downsize. Another mentor, not among those discussed here, responded to one of my articles not with professional insights but with concerns about his heart disease. Tragically, he passed away shortly thereafter. These personal health challenges undoubtedly impact their ability to engage as they once did.

Understanding the disengagement that accompanies aging, retirement, and health challenges allows me to approach my interactions with former mentors with greater empathy and respect. Their concise replies are not a rejection but rather an indication of their current life stage. I am grateful for the time they have given me in the past and the lessons they have imparted, and I respect their need for space.

In reflecting on this experience, I am reminded of the cyclical nature of mentorship. Just as my mentors once guided me, I now find myself in a position to mentor the next generation of physicians. This role comes with its own set of responsibilities and rewards, and I am committed to honoring the legacy of my mentors by providing support and guidance. The legacy of our mentors lives in the countless lives they have touched, and it is our responsibility to continue their work with the same dedication and passion they once embodied.

43. Discordant Harmonies: Medical Leadership Lessons from Famous Musical Breakups

Creative dissonance may splinter medical teams – and iconic songwriting duos.

Nearly 15 years to the day they broke up, Liam and Noel Gallagher, the brothers who form the nucleus of the Britpop band Oasis, announced they are reuniting for a series of concerts in the United Kingdom and Ireland in 2025. Oasis imploded on August 28, 2009, although the Gallagher brothers had a tumultuous relationship for decades. Their relationship has been marred by physical and legal fights, verbal altercations, and their on-again, off-again working dynamic, which kept the band both creatively vibrant and perpetually on the brink of collapse.

I've been thinking about other famous songwriting pairs that have broken up, e.g., Simon & Garfunkel; Lennon & McCartney; Hall & Oates; the Finn Brothers (Neil and Tim); and Ray and Dave Davies of The Kinks. What, if any, implication does the dissolution of these partnerships hold for medical practice?

The breakup of famous singing and songwriting pairs often stems from complex dynamics of creativity, ego, and differing visions. These duos, despite their undeniable musical chemistry, often struggled with balancing individual identities against a shared artistic mission. Over time, creative differences, competition, and personal conflicts strained these relationships to a breaking point.

For instance, Lennon and McCartney's partnership, despite its legendary success, eventually faltered due to artistic divergence and interpersonal tensions, which were exacerbated by external pressures like fame and the business of music. (Contrary to popular notion,

Yoko Ono did not break up the Beatles.) Their disbanding highlights how the balance between collaboration and individual expression can be delicate and easily disrupted.

Neil Finn, the younger yet more celebrated brother of Tim Finn, gradually assumed control of the New Zealand-based band Split Enz, eventually transforming it into the globally successful Crowded House, known for hits like "Don't Dream It's Over." This shift effectively edged Tim out of the spotlight, intensifying the sibling rivalry that had always simmered beneath the surface.

The tension between the Finn brothers, whose last collaborative album was released in 2002, mirrors the infamous discord between Ray and Dave Davies, where jealousy and competition similarly fueled their creative and personal conflicts. Dave's more rebellious and wild nature contrasted with Ray's introspective and controlling demeanor, leading to frequent arguments and even physical altercations.

Another prime example is the Everly Brothers, Phil and Don, whose constant friction over creative control and personal differences led to their acrimonious breakup in 1973. The final straw came during a performance at Knott's Berry Farm, where tensions boiled over, and Phil famously smashed his guitar and stormed off stage, signaling the end of their partnership (they reunited a decade later).

Paul Simon has explained what led to the parting of folk duo Simon & Garfunkel, saying creative tensions and Art Garfunkel's acting career created the "recipe for the breakup of Simon & Garfunkel." Simon was speaking in a 2024 MGM+ documentary series: *In Restless Dreams: The Music of Paul Simon.*

The recent dissolution of Hall & Oates centered on a business dispute, with Hall claiming Oates' actions (to sell his rights to the music) were "the ultimate betrayal" and that Oates was never really his creative partner. They rarely traveled and spent time together over the past 20 years, basically going their separate ways and uniting only for live performances.

In medical practice, we can see these musical dynamics and tensions mirrored in physicians' relationships and between physicians and their teams. Just as creative duos may struggle to maintain harmony, physicians often face challenges in balancing their autonomy with the collaborative demands of healthcare. The pressure to assert individual expertise while also reporting to a department chair or working within a team can lead to friction, much like in the music industry.

The breakup of musical pairs underscores the importance of communication, mutual respect, shared goals, and adaptability in maintaining effective working relationships. All of these are critical in both artistic and medical collaborations. When these elements are lacking, whether in songwriting or in medicine, the result can be a breakdown of the relationship, leading to diminished outcomes.

Moreover, these breakups illustrate the potential dangers of micromanagement (refer to essay 7). In many of these partnerships, one partner might have felt overshadowed or restricted by the other's influence, leading to resentment and eventually a split. This dynamic is especially evident in musical groups where the songwriting pairs are siblings – not only brothers but also sisters.

The duo Heart, comprising Ann and Nancy Wilson, achieved great success together, but underlying creative differences and personal conflicts led them to pursue solo projects and take breaks from their collaboration. Micromanagement and power struggles can thus undermine what may appear to be the strongest partnerships, i.e., those among siblings.

Similarly, in medical practice, when one physician or leader attempts to overly control the work of others, it can stifle innovation, create discord, and hinder the overall effectiveness of the team. For a healthcare team to function optimally, there needs to be a balance between leadership and autonomy, with each member feeling valued and empowered to contribute their best. Just as these musical duos experienced both the heights of collaborative success and the strains of interpersonal conflict, medical professionals must navigate similar dynamics in their work.

Understanding the psychological underpinnings of musical collaborations can inform approaches to medical team cohesion, conflict resolution, and the fostering of a supportive work environment. Moreover, the emotional and psychological impacts of professional separations, akin to those experienced by these musicians, can also resonate with physicians facing the end of long-term collaborations or changes in their professional landscape. Thus, the dissolution of these iconic duos serves as a poignant reminder of the need for resilience, empathy, and proactive relationship management in the medical field.

As an example, consider the relationship between Joseph Murray, MD, and J. Hartwell Harrison, MD. They performed the world's first successful human transplant (a kidney) in 1954. Harrison removed the kidney and Murray transplanted it, conducting their landmark operation between identical twins. Despite their differing roles and areas of expertise – Murray was a plastic surgeon and Harrison was a urologic surgeon – they worked together harmoniously, respecting each other's contributions, which ultimately led to a Nobel Prize in Physiology or Medicine for Murray.

A recent and notable example of successful medical collaboration is the partnership between Katalin Karikó, PhD, and Drew Weissman, MD, PhD. Their pioneering work laid the foundation for the messenger RNA (mRNA) vaccines that played a crucial role in combating COVID-19. In recognition of their groundbreaking research, they were awarded the Nobel Prize in Physiology or Medicine in 2023. Their partnership, characterized by mutual respect and a shared commitment to innovation despite skepticism from the scientific community, led to a revolutionary advancement in vaccine technology that has saved millions of lives worldwide.

Collaboration in both examples exemplifies how a balanced and respectful partnership can lead to significant achievements, whether it's advancing medical science or producing timeless music.

44. Self-Compassion Changes Unhealthy Behaviors

Sustainable changes in health behaviors are achieved one step at a time – and by being kind to yourself.

As a physician, people frequently ask me for advice about their health, but I've struggled to follow my own advice consistently. My weight has fluctuated (mostly upward), my exercise routine has been inconsistent, I over-rely on medication, and I have a serious sweet tooth that's hard to resist. Despite knowing what's best for my health, I often fall short.

Recently, I've noticed a trend among influencers (refer to essays 5 and 6) who promote health through fear, blame, and shame, along with rigid, black-and-white rules. This approach feels unkind and, in my view, deeply unhelpful. Life is not always black and white. Sometimes it can be brutal. Perfect morning routines and deliberate cold exposure advice is meaningless to individuals who may be struggling to get dressed in the morning or find real focus or meaning to their lives.

In working with patients, I've found that empathy, compassion, and meeting people where they are leads to much more meaningful and lasting change. Research supports this, too. Self-compassion doesn't decrease motivation, as some might think; it improves motivation and leads to more sustained behavior change over time. When we treat ourselves with kindness, we're more likely to stay committed to our goals.

Self-compassion is described in the groundbreaking work by Kristin Neff, PhD. It includes three major principles paraphrased here as relevant to health behavior change:

1. **Self-kindness**: being gracious and forgiving of oneself when facing perceived failure rather than being excessively self-critical

2. **Common humanity**: considering one's challenges as profoundly human, not isolating or unique to perceived individual flaws
3. **Mindfulness**: accepting unpleasant experiences as ephemeral, reducing rumination that facilitates depression and reduces motivation, and mitigating self-comparisons.

If a patient is not able to achieve a health goal at first pass, demonstrating self-compassion is critical. After a perceived failure, instead of playing the "shame and blame game," it is more prudent to dig into what barriers arose that made it difficult to achieve the goal in the specified time period. Problem-solve and set goals around *those* factors, including proactively brainstorming and addressing potential future obstacles.

Self-compassion helps individuals focus on the big picture even when specific goals are not achieved. Reducing self-criticism and promoting self-forgiveness can help prevent a small setback (e.g., a missed workout, an unplanned cigarette or extra alcoholic beverage) from leading to resignation, generalization about one's ability to lead a healthy lifestyle, or catastrophic fears that minor deviations from the plan will accelerate the progression of an underlying condition such as cancer or heart disease.

It is critical to normalize and humanize relapses to build scaffolding for greater change over time. This is consistent with the Transtheoretical Model of Change (TTM) developed by James Prochaska, PhD, and associates in the late 1970s. Psychologists found that forming and maintaining healthy habits is an iterative process. The TTM, also known as the Stages of Change Model, is a theoretical framework for understanding how individuals progress through a sequence of stages when modifying behavior. The model identifies six stages through which people typically move:

1. **Precontemplation**: The individual is not yet considering change or is unaware that their behavior is problematic.

2. **Contemplation**: The individual recognizes the problem and begins to think about the possibility of change, weighing the pros and cons.
3. **Preparation**: The individual is planning to take action soon and may start taking small steps toward change.
4. **Action**: The individual actively implements strategies to change their behavior, often requiring significant time and energy.
5. **Maintenance**: The individual works to sustain the new behavior over the long term and prevent relapse.
6. **Termination**: The individual has fully integrated the new behavior into their lifestyle, and the risk of relapse is minimal.

The model also emphasizes that relapse can occur at any stage, and individuals may cycle through the stages multiple times before achieving lasting change. This cyclical nature underscores the complexity and non-linear path of behavior modification.

Successful change comes with small goal-setting, or "one step at a time" mentality. This produces intrinsic reward and self-reinforcement that boosts motivation to take another step forward. With time and progress, significant momentum can be cultivated toward important and sustainable healthy lifestyle change. This approach uses elements of "SMART" goal-setting, originally coined in the business world and later applied to health behavior. "SMART" stands for **S**pecific, **M**easurable, **A**chievable, **R**elevant, and **T**ime-bound.

While I have found this framework helpful in practice, the formation and achievement of SMART goals can be impacted by a lack of self-compassion if a person is unwilling to break down a goal to be appropriately small, specific, realistic, and meaningful to them as an individual. I have found this to be especially true in my work with patients with substance use disorders and the stages they go through as they work towards recovery. Initial relapse is the rule, and it should be viewed as a part of the journey rather than a failure.

The benefit of self-compassion is that it allows individuals to work toward a preventive lifestyle and that goals can be completely tailored to an individual's health status, socioeconomic resources, and intersectional identities (e.g., race/ethnicity/culture, gender, relationship status, etc.). When you combine self-compassion with creativity, most people are able to identify personalized and meaningful ways to pursue a healthier lifestyle and regain their quality of life if faced with a health setback.

There are so many health problems that are lifestyle related. The World Health Organization has estimated that nearly 50% of mortality from such causes could be reduced with healthy behavior regulation – for example, physical inactivity is associated with many chronic diseases, several mental health problems, and difficulty maintaining a healthy weight. Self-compassion as an integral component of self-regulation of health behaviors impacts psychological, emotional, and physical well-being. Such a holistic, non-judgmental view on health is needed and has the potential to revolutionize how society approaches health and behavior.

45. Every Organization Has a Personality

Does yours have a personality disorder?

I've worked for about a dozen healthcare organizations. Every one of them had a personality, shaped by its history, beliefs, behaviors, and leaders. Each company's personality defined its reputation and relationships with customers, partners, and stakeholders. It influenced how employees interacted, made decisions, and approached their work.

The notion that every organization has a distinct personality separate from any individual within that group is founded in Kurt Lewin's work related to group dynamics and applied psychology. Groups, much like individuals, exhibit distinct characteristics and behaviors that define their identity. Both group dynamics and individual behaviors are critical to understanding organizational life.

A tech startup might have a personality that is innovative, flexible, and casual, whereas a traditional financial institution may be more conservative, structured, and formal. Each industry tends to develop its own unique personality based on the nature of its work, the type of people it attracts, and the standards it upholds. Here are a few other examples:

1. **Education**: The education sector typically has a nurturing, inquisitive, and idealistic personality. It is driven by a passion for knowledge, personal growth, and community development. Educators and administrators are often committed to fostering a supportive and stimulating environment for students, encouraging creativity, critical thinking, and lifelong learning.

2. **Retail**: The retail industry tends to have a dynamic, customer-focused, and adaptable personality. It is characterized by a fast-paced environment where trends and consumer preferences can change rapidly. Successful retail organizations prioritize customer satisfaction, innovation in product offerings, and flexibility in operations to stay competitive in the market.
3. **Manufacturing**: Manufacturing often has a practical, process-oriented, and efficiency-driven personality. This industry values precision, reliability, and continuous improvement. Workers and managers in manufacturing are typically focused on optimizing production processes, maintaining high quality standards, and ensuring safety in the workplace.
4. **Hospitality**: The hospitality industry is known for its welcoming, service-oriented, and detail-focused personality. It thrives on creating positive and memorable experiences for guests. Employees in this sector are often skilled in interpersonal communication, problem-solving, and maintaining a high standard of service to ensure customer satisfaction.

The healthcare industry often exhibits a personality that is compassionate, detail-oriented, and resilient. This field attracts individuals who are dedicated to improving the well-being of others and who can handle high-stress situations with empathy and precision. The culture is usually collaborative, as patient care often requires teamwork among various specialists and support staff. I was drawn to health care as much for its character as for its subject matter.

While organizations don't have clinically diagnosed personality disorders, the concept can be metaphorically applied to describe dysfunctional organizational behaviors. When the leadership culture of an organization becomes unhealthy, it can resemble certain characteristics of personality disorders seen in individuals. These dysfunctions can harm the organization's effectiveness, employee morale, and overall reputation. For example:

A **Narcissistic** organization might be overly focused on its own success and image, ignoring the well-being of employees or the needs of customers. This can lead to arrogance, lack of accountability, and a toxic work environment (see essay 47).

A **Paranoid** organization may develop a distrustful atmosphere, with an excessive focus on internal politics, fear of failure, or suspicion of external partners. This can stifle innovation and collaboration.

An **Obsessive-Compulsive** organization could become excessively focused on control, rules, and processes, to the point where flexibility and adaptability are sacrificed, leading to inefficiency and employee burnout.

A **Schizoid** organization might show little to no emotional engagement, operating in a highly isolated manner leading to inefficiencies and a stagnant culture. The organization might appear indifferent to industry standards, social norms, or competitive pressures. The organizational structure can be rigid, with strict hierarchies and little flexibility. It exists in a bubble, often ignoring external feedback. *As I have argued in this book, healthcare systems are dangerously trending in this direction.*

Just as individuals can benefit from increasing self-awareness and modifying their behavior, organizations can achieve significant improvements through interventions aimed at enhancing their overall health and effectiveness. By implementing certain interventions, organizations can make necessary adjustments to their behaviors and strategies. This proactive approach not only helps in addressing any existing issues but also fosters a healthier, more resilient, and more effective organizational environment.

Here are some key interventions that can help organizations address their "personality disorders" and mitigate any negative consequences:

1. **Cultural Transformation**: Organizational culture deeply affects employee morale, productivity, and overall success. When an organization's culture becomes toxic or misaligned with its goals, a cultural transformation may be necessary. This process involves assessing the current culture, identifying desired cultural attributes, and implementing initiatives to bridge the gap. Strategies might include revising core values, enhancing internal communication, recognizing and rewarding desired behaviors, and fostering an inclusive and supportive environment.
2. **Strategic Changes**: Sometimes, the fundamental strategies of an organization need to be reevaluated and adjusted to stay relevant and competitive. This can involve redefining the organization's mission and vision, exploring new market opportunities, diversifying product or service offerings, or optimizing operational processes. Strategic changes require a thorough analysis of the organization's strengths, weaknesses, opportunities, and threats (SWOT analysis), as well as a clear plan for execution and monitoring progress.
3. **Employee Engagement and Development**: Engaged and well-developed employees are essential for a healthy organizational personality. Initiatives to improve employee engagement can include regular feedback mechanisms, professional development opportunities, and creating a sense of purpose and belonging. Encouraging a culture of continuous learning and growth helps employees feel valued and motivated, which in turn positively influences the overall organizational climate.

4. **Change Management**: Successfully navigating organizational change requires a structured approach to managing the transition. Change management practices include clear communication, involving stakeholders in the change process, providing training and support, and addressing resistance. Effective change management ensures that changes are implemented smoothly and that employees are supported throughout the transition, reducing the potential for disruption and dissatisfaction.
5. **Leadership Development**: Effective leadership is crucial for setting the tone and direction of an organization (refer to essay 26). Leadership development programs can help current and future leaders build self-awareness, emotional intelligence, and strategic thinking skills. These programs often include coaching, mentorship, and training in areas such as conflict resolution, decision-making, and effective communication. By investing in leadership development, organizations can cultivate leaders who are capable of inspiring and guiding their teams through change and challenges.

46. Blues Power: Turning Heartache into Healing

This is highly encapsulated but accurate portrayal of the emotional weight of the conversation and the tension between a physician's personal challenges and the desire to heal, both for themselves and their patients.

Patient/Physician (P): I'm an old blues man, and I think that you understand I've been singing the blues ever since the world began.

Psychiatrist (Me): I hear you. That timeless blues spirit runs deep, carrying the weight of lived experience and heartache. It's like a rhythm that never fades, just keeps echoing through every generation. What's got you singing the blues today?

P: Medicine has devolved into a shit show.

Me: I feel that frustration. Medicine has become so entangled in bureaucracy, profit-driven motives, and administrative burdens that it's easy to lose sight of patient care. It's a system where compassion and time are often sacrificed for metrics and margins. What aspects of it feel like the biggest failures to you right now?

P: I don't know where to begin. I just feel so let down by the system. It doesn't work for the benefit of patients or providers.

Me: It's a betrayal, really, when the system that's supposed to heal becomes one that harms – not only patients but those who've dedicated their lives to care for them. When the focus shifts to profits, efficiency, and control, the humanity of medicine fades. Providers are overworked, patients are rushed, and no one feels heard or cared for. What do you think could turn it around? Or at least soften the sharp edges?

P: Honestly, I think it's hopeless. Maybe put more doctors in control of the decisions. Take the administrators and politicians out of the exam room.

Me: That would be a real step in the right direction – letting the people who actually understand patient care, the doctors, guide the system. The problem is that medicine has become too corporate, with too many non-medical folks pulling the strings, turning health care into a commodity. When business decisions overshadow clinical judgment, it's the patients and providers who suffer. It's easy to feel hopeless when it feels like no one's steering the ship with compassion. Do you think there's any way doctors can reclaim some of that control, or is it too far gone?

P: Well, I mentioned that I'm an old bluesman. I actually came of age during the era of rock and roll, and your comment that medicine may be "too far gone" reminds me of the Eagles song "Already Gone." I suppose that's my answer, that in my mind, I've already left it behind. But I don't know what my next step will be. It frightens me, and departing my very sick patients makes me feel guilty.

Me: That makes a lot of sense. Letting go is tough when you've poured so much of yourself into your work, especially when people's lives and well-being are involved. But it sounds like you've given so much already, and the toll this broken system has taken on you is real. "Already Gone" fits the feeling – of knowing it's time to move on, but not without some heartache. Maybe it's not about abandoning your patients, but finding a different way to support them or channel your experience. The path ahead might not be clear yet, but there's still so much you can do, even outside the system. How do you think you might continue to make a difference?

P: Again, your choice of words is uncanny. The Eagles also sang "Heartache Tonight," a romp about getting hurt by staying in a toxic relationship – I'm married to medicine. But to answer your question,

I definitely still feel passionate about the medical field, and I would like to make a contribution, to continue to impact patient care, even if it's through indirect means. Do you have any suggestions?

Me: I'm glad to hear that passion for medicine is still alive in you – it can be channeled in ways that bring fulfillment without being caught up in the mess of the system. Here are a few ideas on how you could make an impact indirectly:

1. **Teaching and Mentorship**: Sharing your knowledge with younger physicians or medical students could shape the next generation of compassionate, patient-centered doctors. You can pass on the values you feel the system is missing.
2. **Writing and Advocacy**: You're a capable writer judging by your publications. Maybe you could become a voice for change through writing or public speaking, shedding light on the systemic issues while advocating for reforms that put patient care first.
3. **Volunteering**: There are many opportunities to use your expertise in non-profit organizations, free clinics, or community health initiatives that don't have the same bureaucratic weight as hospitals and large systems.
4. **Consulting**: Your experience could be invaluable in advising health care organizations or startups on how to create patient-centered systems or improve current practices.
5. **Public Health**: This is a fantastic avenue for making a broad impact! It focuses on improving health outcomes for communities and populations, which aligns perfectly with your desire to contribute meaningfully.
6. **Telemedicine or Specialty Care**: You might still be able to see patients in a more controlled, flexible environment through telemedicine or by offering second opinions or specialty consultations that don't involve the same administrative burden.

Do any of these resonate with where you're at?

P: Actually, all of these options are appealing. I just don't know how to get started. Also, I've been thinking about working as a locum tenens physician. I've read positive stories about this type of work.

Me: It's great that all those options resonate with you – it shows that you've got a lot of potential paths forward. Locum tenens work could be a solid bridge, too, giving you the chance to continue practicing while having more control over your schedule and environment. To get started with each of these options, here's a breakdown:

1. **Locum Tenens**: There are several agencies that specialize in locum tenens placements. You could start by researching reputable agencies (CompHealth, Weatherby Healthcare, or LocumTenens.com) to find a good fit. Many of them offer flexible opportunities that might allow you to explore other interests alongside practicing medicine. Talk to other physicians who have worked locum tenens to get their perspective and advice.
2. **Teaching/Mentorship**: Reach out to medical schools, residency programs, or even online platforms like Coursera or MedEd platforms where you could contribute as a lecturer or mentor. Consider joining professional organizations that have mentorship programs, or look for conferences that offer opportunities to teach workshops.
3. **Writing/Advocacy**: Perhaps starting a blog or contributing op-eds to medical journals or mainstream publications could be the next step. Advocacy groups often look for people with your kind of experience to help frame important issues. Joining professional networks or organizations that focus on health care reform or patient advocacy could give you a platform to push for change.
4. **Volunteering**: Look into organizations like Doctors Without Borders, local free clinics, or national medical outreach

programs. Many allow for short-term or flexible commitments that align with your skills and experience.

5. **Consulting**: You could begin by offering pro bono advice to healthcare startups or non-profits, then build your reputation and expand your network. Platforms like LinkedIn are great for showcasing your expertise and connecting with companies in need of medical insight.
6. **Public Health**: Getting started in public health can often involve networking with professionals in the field, attending workshops or conferences, and finding volunteer opportunities to gain experience. You can get involved through public health departments and community health initiatives, non-profit foundations, and global health organizations.

Locum tenens could also give you time to explore these indirect paths without fully committing to one right away.

P: That sounds great. Thanks for your advice. Same time next week?

Me: Why? There's no point in crying the blues anymore!

47. Leaving a Toxic Company – And Preparing for One Less Toxic

Anticipate difficult questions during your job interview, but control the narrative.

Many years ago, I left an organization that was extremely toxic. It was causing me to become depressed. During my exit interview, I was asked by a representative from human resources (HR) why I hadn't come forth earlier. She said she would have conducted a "climate assessment." A climate assessment takes the temperature of an organization and provides leadership with feedback by identifying areas of strength and those in need of improvement.

I was unaware such a mechanism was available to me. Instead, I clung to my job despite its toxic effects. I later learned from a physician who had previously held the same position that he, too, became clinically depressed. The source of our distress was our boss whom we both felt had a severe personality disorder. Toxic bosses harm employees in countless ways, and estimates suggest abusive supervision costs organizations millions in lost productivity, employee turnover, and litigation each year.

In rare instances, the behaviors of toxic leaders can "trickle down" to affect the actions of employees at lower organizational levels, resulting in abused supervisors who abuse their own subordinates, much like the cycle of abuse seen in families. However, research shows that people who disidentify with their toxic boss are less likely to adopt bad behavior – especially when the person has high integrity and morals.

My upfront advice is to learn how to read the tea leaves and quickly depart any company that is making you sick. It took more than 100 doctors and faculty members at the University of Virginia

(UVA) School of Medicine and health system to highlight the toxic working conditions there. They signed a no-confidence letter (dated September 5, 2024) against two physician administrators: K. Craig Kent, MD, UVA Health's CEO and executive vice president for health affairs, and Melina Kibbe, MD, dean of the school of medicine. The letter included allegations over concerns about patient safety, such as quality of new doctor hires; fear of retaliation against those who raise concerns about patient safety, capacity constraints, and moral distress; excessive spending on C-suite executives amid staffing shortages; and failure to be forthcoming on significant financial matters. The letter also mentioned that the environment fostered by Drs. Kent and Kibbe has contributed "to an ongoing exodus of experience and expertise at all levels."

Such displays of unison among faculty are rare. It is more typical of physicians to hold on to toxic jobs or work for toxic bosses to the point where it is affecting their health. This is usually due to a combination of financial, professional, and psychological factors. Financially, the significant investment in medical education and training, coupled with the high costs of student loans, can make the prospect of leaving a steady job daunting.

Professionally, physicians may fear damaging their reputation or career trajectory by leaving a position prematurely, especially in a field where relationships and networks are crucial. Additionally, the deeply ingrained culture of resilience and dedication in medicine can lead physicians to endure adverse conditions, believing it's their duty to persevere for the sake of their patients. Furthermore, toxic leaders may manipulate or undermine physicians' confidence, making them feel trapped or incapable of finding better opportunities.

Lastly, the scarcity of job openings in certain specialties or geographic locations can limit options, compelling physicians to stay in less-than-ideal work environments. These intertwined factors create a complex scenario where physicians might remain in toxic settings despite the personal and professional toll it takes on them.

Assuming you find your situation intolerable and decide to move on, whatever feelings you may harbor about the people in your organization should not carry over into a prospective job interview and new position. Complaining about your former boss or coworkers especially in an interview is a big mistake. You must navigate a job interview after leaving a toxic workplace with grace and professionalism. It can be tricky.

Here's an example of how you might respond to a question about why you left (or are planning to leave) your job:

"While I appreciated the opportunities I had at my previous job, I realized that I was looking for a work environment that better aligns with my professional values and career goals. I am excited about the opportunity at your company because it offers the kind of collaborative and supportive culture where I believe I can thrive and make significant contributions."

Here are some short-answer options for responding to that same time-honored question:

Q: Why are you leaving?
A: "There's been a mismatch in expectations." Or, "I'm looking for a role where I can learn and be challenged." Or, "It wasn't a good fit for me."

Sometimes it's best to keep it simple. Above all, never say anything negative. Save your rants for your therapist or coach.

You'll likely face other challenging questions during your new job interview. Don't allow yourself to get tripped up by them. Stick to the facts and remain neutral. You will have the ability to control the narrative to some extent. Hook people in. Tell them your story in a way that captures their attention from the get-go. Remember, this isn't the dust jacket bio of your book; it's your chance to introduce yourself to the interviewer.

For example:
Q: Why are you leaving so soon (assume less than three years)?
A: "I saw the job description (online, etc.), and it's a better fit for me than my current job. Here's what resonates with me…"

During the interview, highlight specific skills you've gained: "I'm looking to deepen my interests in IT and forecasting."

Highlight your values: "I'm seeking a company that respects teamwork and collaboration."

Emphasize your strengths: "I'm a fast learner and quickly adapt to new situations."

Research the company and show that you're a good cultural fit: "I'm looking forward to working with the chief medical officer and her team. They've demonstrated novel approaches to patient care."

Share what's important to you: "I'm looking forward to celebrating our wins."

Tell the interviewer what you have learned: "I've become deeply passionate about public health and patient advocacy."

Take the focus off of a negative topic. "My colleagues swear by my character and work ethic (playful yet serious). I've listed them as references."

Shift to your ambitions and express enthusiasm: "I'm eager to join a team that values creativity and innovation."

Talk about your professional development: “I’m seeking a company that invests in its employees’ education.”

Show growth from adversity: “I’m sure I can make a positive contribution.”

Lastly, don’t be afraid to show yourself and spotlight what you do outside of working hours: “I volunteer once a month at a free clinic.” Or, “I play the piano (or other instrument).” Or, “I enjoy writing poetry.” By law, they can’t ask personal issues, and I would recommend that you avoid raising them, e.g., family, culture, religion, sexual preference, and political and ideological affiliations and positions.

Looking back on my situation, I’m not so sure a climate assessment would have done any good, because giving feedback seemed tantamount to the proverbial fox guarding the henhouse: it takes courageous leaders to recognize their faults and seek help when they need it. In the case of UVA, a public information officer said that the health system’s leadership is looking to further examine faculty members’ concerns and that the organization values feedback from its employees. But if they are not motivated to change their ways and the corporate culture, the feedback is useless, or worse yet, may be used in retaliation.

Nevertheless, I think there is a responsibility to provide *constructive* feedback to an organization that is in the habit of taking its temperature and is sincere about doing something when it is high. If they are not genuine in their offer to make changes or accommodations, you may be forced to leave your job no matter how much you enjoy it. There is no point in staying at a job you love if the conditions all around you scream that your well-being is at risk.

Leaving a toxic job may not be easy, but your experience can make you a stronger candidate. By preparing in advance and maintaining a positive, professional demeanor, you can navigate a new job interview successfully and leave a strong impression on your potential employer. Anticipate challenging questions during the interview, but control the narrative. Remember, every ending is a new beginning. Own your story and let it elevate you.

48. The Worst Career Advice I Ever Received

It wasn't "plastics."

Do you remember the classic 1967 film *The Graduate*? Dustin Hoffman's character, Benjamin Braddock, receives a piece of career advice that becomes iconic: "Plastics."

I was told that if I shifted from clinical practice to clinical management, I could grow my career. This has to the worst piece of advice I ever received – not because it's not true, but because not everyone thrives in management. This is especially true of physicians who prefer to delegate administrative duties and remain in the safe, clinical confines of practice, shielded from operations and logistics. Clinical managers tend to work extra-long hours and are saddled with tons of projects and daily administrative activities. As a manager, you'll need to make significant sacrifices, dole out bad news to people, and manage some who are incorrigible.

One of my first tasks as the medical director of a psychiatric hospital was to respond to a nurse who roared into my office. "Dr Lazarus," she exclaimed with a look of exasperation that caused me to dread what came next, "I went to see Dr. Merkel (not his real name). He was in his office, sitting behind his desk, bare-chested, just staring out into space. What should we do?"

I was not the least bit prepared or inclined to handle this situation, but as medical director, the responsibility fell on me. Dealing with bizarre psychiatric patients is part-and-parcel of what we do as psychiatrists. But dealing with bizarre colleagues is a whole other matter and not for everyone. Rather than take on the high stress that comes with executive positions, I was content to assume roles in middle management. I never missed having "CEO" attached to my name.

You are bound to receive lots of career advice, some of which may be outdated or counterproductive. One common piece of advice that should be reconsidered is the notion that you should always prioritize work over personal life. While dedication and hard work are essential in the medical field, maintaining a healthy work-life balance is crucial for long-term success and personal well-being. It has been shown that over-worked, unwell physicians negatively impact healthcare systems by affecting recruitment and retention of physicians, workplace productivity and efficiency, and quality of patient care and patient safety.

Physicians are told to “follow the money” and leave their passions for their hobbies. But that’s a trap, because prioritizing salary over job satisfaction will eventually result in resentment and lack of motivation. A smarter move is to align financial rewards with pursuing work that you find meaningful. Build on your passions to develop rare and valuable skills that you can market to employers. The corollary is “don’t let your salary be a liability.” In other words, be content with a compensation package in the mid-range for your specialty (refer to essay 25). Asking for a top-level salary may peg you as a demanding or unreasonable person.

However, the notion that you should avoid discussing financial aspects of your practice is not true. Financial literacy is an important aspect of managing a medical career, whether you are in private practice or an employee of a large healthcare organization. Understanding the financial operations, reimbursement processes, and economic challenges of the healthcare system can empower you to make informed decisions that benefit your practice and patients.

Another outdated suggestion is that you should stick rigidly to traditional career paths within your specialty. The medical field is rapidly evolving, and opportunities in areas like telemedicine, consulting, and research are expanding (refer to essay 46). You should feel empowered to explore these non-traditional roles if they align better with your skills and interests. Diversifying your career can lead to more fulfilling professional experiences and can also contribute to the broader healthcare landscape in innovative ways. My career has been interesting because it has been diverse, marked by both traditional and non-traditional jobs.

The advice to avoid seeking help or admitting uncertainty can be detrimental. Medicine is a collaborative field, and acknowledging the limits of your knowledge is a strength, not a weakness. Seeking mentorship, participating in continuous education, and consulting with colleagues are vital practices that enhance professional growth and improve patient outcomes. Embracing a culture of learning and humility can lead to more effective and compassionate medical practice.

Physicians are often told to "fake it 'til you make it," which is wrong. Faking situations in life can backfire, leading to mistakes and loss of credibility. You should be honest about your knowledge gaps and seek learning opportunities to fill them. Project confidence, yet actively work to increase your expertise. Remember, hard work alone does not always pay off. In fact, insistence on hard work as a guarantee of success is another piece of bad advice. Success is *never* guaranteed.

Many of us are admonished to keep our heads down and do our work. This, too, is bad advice. The lack of visibility will hinder your career growth. Show initiative and seek out new projects. Networking and visibility are key to career advancement.

Finally, you can say "no" to your boss, contrary to opinion that you should never say "no" to her. Always saying "yes" can lead to more work and burnout. Your opinions may be undervalued if you simply say "yes" to everything. There are no doubt times when your boss doesn't know the answer to a problem or may be testing you, hoping you have the courage to disagree with him. There is nothing wrong with politely asserting yourself to people in authority. The historian and author Doris Kearns Goodwin famously said, "Good leadership requires you to surround yourself with people of diverse perspectives who can disagree with you without fear of retaliation."

Take control of your career by making informed choices. Don't let outmoded advice hold you back. Critically evaluate any career advice you receive and be open to modern perspectives that promote balance, innovation, collaboration, and financial acumen. By doing so, you can forge a career path that is not only successful but also personally and professionally fulfilling.

49. Embracing Psychiatry as a Specialty

The growing appeal of psychiatry for medical graduates and the rewards of a career in mental health.

In recent years, there has been a noticeable trend of more medical school graduates choosing to enter the field of psychiatry. A total of 1,746 U.S. medical school graduates – 1,343 from allopathic schools and 403 from osteopathic schools – matched into psychiatry residency programs in 2023 as part of the National Resident Matching Program (NRMP). It marks the 12th year in a row that psychiatry's match numbers have increased.

This shift can be attributed to a growing recognition of mental health's critical role in overall well-being and the increasing societal acceptance of seeking help for mental health issues. As awareness and de-stigmatization of mental health conditions improve, more graduates are drawn to psychiatry, inspired by the opportunity to make a significant and positive impact on patients' lives.

In fact, a 2023 study published in the journal *BMC Medical Education* showed that more than half of medical students have a change of heart about their specialty choice during their four-year journey to starting residency. From a sample of more than 10,000 students, 56% changed their career choice between their second year of medical school and graduation, and of those, the specialty toward which most students switched their choice was psychiatry, with a 172% rise in students preferring the field.

The specialty that remained the most consistent choice among students between their second year and graduation was also psychiatry. More than 70% of students who preferred psychiatry as second-year medical students listed it as their choice at the time of graduation. (Other specialties that had high retention from the second year to graduation were family medicine [65.1%], anesthesia [58.5%], emergency medicine [56.1%] and pediatrics [56.1%].)

The study did not explore the reasons why psychiatry was a highly preferred specialty, but it did note that many characteristics, including future salary, the competitiveness of the field, and the importance of work-life balance, were significantly associated with a higher likelihood of changing career choices in general. In my experience, medical students are typically drawn to psychiatry by a desire to help those struggling with mental health issues and to explore the intricate interplay between biological, psychological, and social factors that influence mental health – the so-called "biopsychosocial" model of treatment.

The term "biopsychosocial" was coined by George L. Engel, MD, in 1977. Engel, an internist and psychiatrist, introduced this holistic approach to understanding and treating illness, emphasizing the interconnection between biological, psychological, and social factors in health and disease. His seminal paper, "The Need for a New Medical Model: A Challenge for Biomedicine," published in the journal *Science*, laid the foundation for this comprehensive framework.

Engel wrote, "The dominant model of disease today [1970s] is biomedical, and it leaves no room within its framework for the social, psychological, and behavioral dimensions of illness. A biopsychosocial model is proposed that provides a blueprint for research, a framework for teaching, and a design for action in the real world of health care."

This model was ingrained in me throughout my medical school education (1976-1980) and residency training (1980-1984). I was stationed all of those years at Temple University School of Medicine, where a handful of psychiatric faculty members had trained under Engel and his associate, John Romano, MD, at the University of

Rochester School of Medicine. (The Rochester-Temple connection persists today through a drug discovery partnership.)

The biopsychosocial model has since become a cornerstone in various medical and psychological disciplines, promoting a more integrated and patient-centered approach to care. Its universal appeal attracts students who are usually motivated by a combination of intellectual curiosity and a commitment to patient-centered care, finding the prospect of building long-term therapeutic relationships particularly rewarding. Individuals in alignment with the biopsychosocial model often gravitate toward careers in psychiatry and family medicine. They possess a deep empathy and a genuine interest in the wonders of the human mind and the interface between mental and physical health and disease.

Psychiatry allows for a diverse range of practice settings, from private practice to hospitals and community health centers, providing flexibility and variety in professional life. Additionally, psychiatrists have the opportunity to engage in various therapeutic modalities, such as psychotherapy, pharmacotherapy ("medication management"), and emerging treatments like neuromodulation. The continuous advancements in understanding mental health and developing new treatments also ensure that psychiatry remains an intellectually stimulating and dynamic specialty. For those passionate about making a real difference in the lives of individuals and communities, psychiatry offers a deeply rewarding and enriching career.

Unfortunately, about half of medical schools do not begin their core clinical clerkship rotations until students enter their third year of medical school, meaning many have limited specialty exposure. As I explored my career options, my rotations proved to be a key selling point. When I started my clerkships, I was predisposed toward psychiatry – I majored in psychology during college – and it did, in fact, become my calling. No other rotation except neurology held as much appeal. However, the key takeaway is that gaining clinical experience and interacting with patients in their environment was far more valuable for me in identifying my interests than any preconceived notions I had from college.

My advice to medical students, whether they change their specialty choice or stick with their original plans, is to follow your passions. Pick a specialty based on what type of clinical environment makes you excited to come to work every day, where you feel most comfortable, where you seem excited about types of the cases that you'll be seeing, and where nothing seems like a chore, even if it is the least exciting part of the job. If you can deal with that element of the job – aspects that excite you least – then maybe that specialty is right for you, even if it's not psychiatry!

50. Live Long and Die Short

It's not about adding years to life; it's about adding life to years.

Americans want to grow old in their own homes. But pursuing that dream has gotten harder, and is putting huge financial and emotional strains on families who face soaring costs and mounting pressures in taking care of their loved ones. It's indisputable that the costs of aging at home can have enormous effects on a family's financial security, health and quality of life. But for anyone who needed a reminder, a 2024 *Wall Street Journal* article, "The Crushing Financial Burden of Aging at Home," provided a searing reality check.

In Nebraska, Christine Salhany spends about $240,000 a year for a team of five people to provide 24-hour in-home care for her husband who has Alzheimer's disease. In Illinois, Carolyn Brugioni's father exhausted his savings and took out a home-equity line-of-credit to pay for home healthcare. Many other families lose sleep, put their lives on hold and drain their savings when an older loved one needs in-home care.

Some adults in their 50s and 60s look toward the future and say, "I'll just age in place. It's cheaper. When my spouse or I need care, we can stay home and take care of each other."

Similarly, many adult children of older parents assume they can arrange care for mom and dad at their home when the need arises. What they don't realize is that aging in place without a realistic plan is a bad idea. It takes real foresight and sometimes a village (and significant financial resources) to enable loved ones to live at home safely and productively longer. The best way to do that is to increase investment in healthy longevity.

Over a decade ago, a landmark ten-year study by the MacArthur Foundation shattered the stereotypes of aging as a process of slow, genetically determined decline. Researchers found that 70% of physical aging, and about 50% of mental aging, is determined by lifestyle, the choices we make every day. Additional research showed that people who live longer often experience shorter periods of decline before death, a phenomenon sometimes referred to as "compression of morbidity." That means that if we optimize healthy lifestyles, we can "live longer and die shorter," i.e., condense the decline period into the very end of a fulfilling, active old age.

Some studies do not support compression of morbidity when morbidity is defined as major disease and mobility functioning loss. However, whether or not the concept is valid, no one can argue that living longer and dying shorter emphasizes the goal of maintaining good health and quality of life for as long as possible in order to minimize prolonged suffering or chronic illness. Living long and dying short is a concept that underscores the importance of not only extending one's lifespan but also ensuring that the years lived are marked by health and vitality with minimal burden placed upon loved ones. Achieving this ideal involves a multifaceted approach that encompasses physical, mental, and emotional well-being.

Maintaining physical health is paramount. This involves regular exercise, which helps in managing weight, improving cardiovascular health, and boosting overall energy levels. A balanced diet rich in fruits, vegetables, whole grains, and lean proteins provides the necessary nutrients for the body to function optimally. Regular medical check-ups and screenings are essential to detect and address potential health issues early, preventing them from developing into more serious conditions. Additionally, avoiding harmful habits such as smoking and excessive alcohol consumption can significantly reduce the risk of chronic diseases.

Mental health is equally important in the quest to live long and die short. Engaging in activities that stimulate the mind, such as reading, puzzles, or learning new skills, can help maintain cognitive function. Social connections play a crucial role in mental well-being;

maintaining strong relationships with family, friends, and community can provide emotional support and reduce feelings of loneliness and depression. Stress management techniques, such as mindfulness, meditation, and yoga, can also help in maintaining mental equilibrium.

Emotional well-being is another critical component. Finding purpose and meaning in life, whether through work, hobbies, or volunteering, can provide a sense of fulfillment and satisfaction. Practicing gratitude and maintaining a positive outlook can enhance emotional resilience, helping individuals to cope better with life's challenges. It is also important to seek help when needed, whether through therapy, counseling, or support groups, to address emotional issues and maintain overall well-being. Overcoming Erikson's "integrity versus despair" stage of life (>65 years) means you have resolved the key conflict of questioning whether or not you have led a meaningful, satisfying life.

Lastly, adopting a proactive approach to aging can help ensure that the later years are lived with quality. This might involve making necessary adjustments to living environments to ensure safety and accessibility, staying engaged in social and community activities, and continuing to pursue passions and interests. By focusing on preventive care and maintaining a healthy lifestyle, individuals can reduce the duration and severity of decline at the end of life.

Living long and dying short is about more than just adding years to life; it's about adding life to years. Through a combination of physical health, mental stimulation, emotional well-being, and proactive aging, individuals can strive to live vibrant, fulfilling lives, minimizing the period of decline and ensuring a dignified end without burdening families. Here are a few pointers to keep in mind as society collectively strives to reach that goal:

- Recognize just how expensive the unplanned alternative is, i.e., reactive, after-the-fact, aging at home.

- Empower older adults to take charge of their health and proactively manage their chronic conditions before they're in need of round-the-clock care. Engage those who express disinterest in routine care and medical exams.
- Offer alternative viewpoints to fatalistic attitudes and perceptions that view declining health is an inevitable part of aging.
- Educate older adults who might feel overwhelmed by the complexity of modern health care, preferring to rely on familiar, albeit outdated, practices.
- Strengthen systems of preventive and predictive health care. Public health campaigns should emphasize the importance of regular check-ups, highlighting success stories of older adults who have benefited from proactive health measures.
- Encourage people in their 40s, 50s and 60s to adopt the healthy lifestyles that will allow them to avoid or at least delay loss of mobility or cognitive function. What we used to think of as diseases of aging, such as high blood pressure, atherosclerosis, heart attacks and cancer, we now see in people as young as 20.

If we take the right steps, many more Baby Boomers and Gen-Xers will have the opportunity to "live long and die short." More older adults will have the opportunity to age gracefully and die with dignity rather than spend 10 or 15 years of progressive, debilitating, and costly decline. Older adults need to become more proactive in planning for their future. They need to seize the opportunity now.

AFTERWORD

51. Opportunity Costs Manifest Near Retirement

Final reflections on a life well lived.

This book may well be my last, not due to any decline in health or imminent peril, but because I have shared nearly everything from my life and career that I believe holds value and lessons for readers. The pages of this book contain the final pieces of my story, both literally and figuratively. Now in semi-retirement, I spend my winters in Hawaii, embracing the opportunity to truly stop and smell the flowers. Aloha 'Oe to the chapters of my life that have been written and shared across six volumes.

Though I might continue to write and publish essays online, the originality of those future works may not match the freshness of this volume and my previous ones. There comes a point when a person has expressed all their thoughts and ideas, and the novelty begins to fade, much like an old pair of jeans – still comfortable but no longer new. Borrowing from Jerry Garcia, I don't want to go down the road feeling bad, or be seen as a writer over the hill. I would rather stop while I'm ahead than risk diminishing my legacy by overstaying my creative peak, much like athletes who continue beyond their prime.

In this book, recognizing it might be my last, I have endeavored to encapsulate the essence of my experiences, insights, and the wisdom I have gathered over the years. Each essay is a piece of my heart, a fragment of my journey, and a testament to the moments that have shaped me. I hope that readers find value in these stories and reflections, as they are the culmination of a life lived with passion, curiosity, and a relentless pursuit of understanding.

Semi-retirement has afforded me the luxury of time – time to reflect, to savor the present, and to embrace the tranquility that comes with a life no longer bound by deadlines and demands. In Hawaii, I find relaxation in the rhythm of the waves, the vibrant hues of the sunsets, and the gentle sway of the palm trees. It is here that I have come to appreciate the beauty of simplicity and the profound joy of living in the moment.

As I gradually step away from the fray of professional life, I am reminded of the importance of balance and the need to nurture one's spirit. Writing has been my outlet, my means of processing the world around me, and sharing my thoughts with others. While this book may mark the end of an era, it also signifies a new beginning – a chapter where I can explore other facets of life that I may have overlooked in the hustle and bustle of my career.

The concept of "opportunity cost" from economics can provide a valuable framework for understanding the personal value system of a physician who is nearing the end of their career, considering retirement, or contemplating an encore career. Opportunity cost refers to the benefits an individual misses out on when choosing one alternative over another. For a seasoned physician, this concept can help elucidate the trade-offs involved in their decision-making processes at this critical juncture in their professional life.

As I approach retirement, the opportunity cost of continuing employment might be measured against the potential benefits of spending more time with family, pursuing personal interests, or engaging in leisure activities. For instance, if I decide to extend my career by a few more years, I might miss valuable opportunities to travel with my wife, engage in hobbies I have long set aside (mainly listening to and playing music), or simply enjoy the freedom of an unstructured day. The satisfaction derived from these personal pursuits could be a significant factor in my decision to retire, underscoring the value I place on personal fulfillment and quality of life outside of my professional identity.

On the other hand, if I consider an encore career, perhaps in medical education, the opportunity cost involves weighing the benefits of continued professional engagement against the potential loss of the relaxed lifestyle that retirement offers. For example, transitioning into a role as a mentor, coach, and teacher might provide me with intellectual stimulation, a sense of purpose, and the opportunity to impart my accumulated knowledge to the next generation of physicians and psychiatrists. However, this choice also means sacrificing the complete freedom and reduced stress levels that come with full retirement. The decision hinges on whether the intrinsic rewards of continued professional involvement outweigh the allure of a more leisurely lifestyle.

Ultimately, the personal value system of a physician, shaped by a lifetime of dedication to patient welfare, professional growth, and personal sacrifices, will play a crucial role in navigating these opportunity costs. The decision to retire, continue practicing, or embark on an encore career involves a complex interplay of professional satisfaction, personal fulfillment, and the desire to make a lasting impact. By understanding the opportunity costs associated with each option, I can make a well-informed decision that aligns with my values and aspirations for the future.

I find it interesting that unlike past generations of retirees who generally stopped working at retirement, the next generation saving for retirement seems less eager to relax once they leave their 9-to-5 job. Just 11% of would-be retirees surveyed by CNBC in August 2024 say they don't plan to work in any capacity after they retire. More than a third of respondents – 36% – say they're not sure, while the majority, 53%, anticipate working, either because they'll want to or to supplement their income.

Whatever the next chapter holds – even if there is not another book "chapter" – to my readers I extend my deepest gratitude. Your support, feedback, and shared experiences have enriched my journey and fueled my desire to write. It is my hope that my words have resonated with you, offered solace during difficult times, and inspired you to pursue your own passions with fervor and determination.

I leave you with this thought: Life is an ever-evolving narrative, a tapestry woven with threads of joy, sorrow, triumph, and failure. Embrace each chapter with an open heart and an inquisitive mind. Cherish the lessons learned and the memories made. And never underestimate the power of your own story.

Thank you for allowing me to share mine. Aloha and farewell – for now.

About the Author

Arthur L. Lazarus, MD, MBA, is a healthcare consultant, certified physician executive, and nationally recognized author, speaker, and champion of physician leadership and wellness. He has broad experience in clinical practice and the health insurance industry, having led programs at Cigna and Humana. At Humana, Lazarus was vice president and corporate medical director of behavioral health operations in Louisville, Kentucky, and subsequently a population health medical director in the state of Florida.

Lazarus has also held leadership positions in several pharmaceutical companies, including Pfizer and AstraZeneca, conducting clinical trials, and reviewing promotional material for medical accuracy and FDA compliance. He has published more than 400 articles and essays online and in scientific and professional journals and has written and edited ten books, including six related to the field of narrative medicine.

Born in Philadelphia, Pennsylvania, Lazarus attended Boston University, where he graduated with a bachelor's degree in psychology with Distinction. He received his medical degree with Honors from Temple University School of Medicine, followed by a psychiatric residency at Temple University Hospital, where he was chief resident. After residency, Lazarus joined the faculty of Temple University School of Medicine, where he currently serves as Adjunct Professor of Psychiatry. He also holds non-faculty appointments as Executive-in-Residence at Temple University Fox School of Business and Management, where he received his MBA degree, and Senior Fellow, Jefferson College of Population Health, Philadelphia, Pennsylvania.

Well known for his leadership and medical management skills, Lazarus is a sought-after presenter, mentor, teacher, and writer. He has shared his expertise and perspective at numerous local, national, and international meetings and seminars.

Lazarus is a past president of the American Association for Psychiatric Administration and Leadership, a former member of the board of directors of the American Association for Physician Leadership (AAPL), and a current member of the AAPL editorial review board. In 2010, the American Psychiatric Association honored Lazarus with the Administrative Psychiatry Award for his effectiveness as an administrator of major mental health programs and expanding the body of knowledge of management science in mental health services delivery systems.

Lazarus is among a select group of physicians in the United States who have been inducted into both the Alpha Omega Alpha medical honor society and the Beta Gamma Sigma honor society of collegiate schools of business.

Lazarus enjoys walking, biking, playing piano, and listening to music. He has been happily married to his wife, Cheryl, for over 40 years. They are the proud parents of four adult children and the grandparents of five young children.

Notes

Prologue/Essay 1

1. *Rolling Stone* review, "King Crimson's '21st Century Schizoid Man': Inside Prog's Big Bang": https://www.rollingstone.com/music/music-features/king-crimson-interview-writing-21st-century-schizoid-man-891600/
2. The Commonwealth Fund, "Private Equity's Role in Heath Care": https://www.commonwealthfund.org/publications/explainer/2023/nov/private-equity-role-health-care
3. *JAMA* article: https://jamanetwork.com/journals/jama/article-abstract/2813379
4. Nash DB. "Creating a 'Healthier' Health System: How Hard Could It Be?": https://www.medpagetoday.com/opinion/focusonpolicy/112153
5. *The Commonwealth Fund* report, "Mirror, Mirror 2024: A Portrait of the Failing U.S. Health System": https://www.commonwealthfund.org/publications/fund-reports/2024/sep/mirror-mirror-2024

Essay 4

1. AMA report on burnout: https://www.ama-assn.org/practice-management/physician-health/burnout-falls-still-hits-these-6-physician-specialties-most

Essay 6

1. Serena Williams/Ubrelvy TV ad: https://www.fda.gov/media/181754/download?attachment

Essay 7

1. "Impact of Organizational Leadership on Physician Burnout and Satisfaction": https://documents.christianacare.org/medical-dental%20staff/2015-Impact_of_Organizational_Leadership_on_Physician.pdf

Essay 8

1. Cox small business survey on the impact of AI: https://www.coxblue.com/SmallBizSurvey/

Essay 11

1. FDA guidance documents: https://www.fda.gov/regulatory-information/search-fda-guidance-documents

Essay 14

1. Levine quote: https://www.theguardian.com/politics/2021/dec/28/rachel-levine-us-trans-health-official-profile
2. Fauci quote: https://www.medpagetoday.com/special-reports/heavy-hitters/111242

Essay 18

1. *Annals of Internal Medicine*: https://www.acpjournals.org/doi/10.7326/M23-3475

Essay 19

1. *Journal of Preventive Medicine & Public Health*: https://www.jpmph.org/journal/view.php?doi=10.3961/jpmph.14.031

Essay 20

1. Harvard study of CTE in American football players: https://jamanetwork.com/journals/jamaneurology/fullarticle/2824064

Essay 21

1. Family medicine physician article and quote: https://www.aafp.org/pubs/fpm/issues/2013/0100/p21.html
2. Use of email by older adults: https://www.jmir.org/2009/2/e18/PDF
3. Trends in mental health diagnosis/conditions: https://s3.amazonaws.com/media2.fairhealth.org/whitepaper/asset/Trends%20in%20Mental%20Health%20Conditions%20-%20A%20FAIR%20Health%20White%20Paper.pdf

Essay 22

1. *BMJ* "expression of concern": https://www.bmj.com/content/385/bmj.q1025
2. Alleged abuse of study participants: https://www.theguardian.com/world/2022/jun/20/mdma-trials-canada-review-alleged-abuse
3. *Psychopharmacology* retraction notice: https://link.springer.com/article/10.1007/s00213-024-06665-y

Essay 23

1. AMA survey: https://www.ama-assn.org/system/files/prior-authorization-survey.pdf
2. AMA Leadership Viewpoints: https://www.ama-assn.org/about/leadership/we-must-fix-prior-authorization-protect-our-patients

Essay 23

1. Orthopedic case report: https://www.kevinmd.com/2024/08/why-doctors-are-afraid-to-take-on-insurance-giants-and-how-it-hurts-patients.html
2. *JAMA* article on evidence-based medicine: https://jamanetwork.com/journals/jama/fullarticle/1104225

Essay 25

1. Top CEO salaries at healthcare nonprofits: https://www.erieri.com/blog/post/top-10-highest-paid-ceos-at-nonprofits
2. Executive greed: https://www.bloomberg.com/opinion/articles/2024-07-25/steward-health-bankruptcy-is-a-case-study-in-executive-greed?srnd=all
3. Top CEO salaries at public companies in Seattle, Washington: https://www.seattletimes.com/business/see-how-new-boeing-chief-kelly-ortbergs-pay-compares-with-was-best-paid-ceos/
4. *Health Affairs* article: https://www.healthaffairs.org/content/forefront/non profit-hospital-ceo-compensation-much-enough

Essay 27

1. Family medicine physician article: https://www.doximity.com/articles/688a029e-69dc-4824-ac71-a7dcdcaa674a?clicked=true&cme_search_term_id=280324&position=13&source=search
2. Harris poll: https://www.athenahealth.com/press-releases/us-physicians-surveyed-feel-burned-out-on-a-regular-basis
3. Elsevier Health survey: https://www.elsevier.com/promotions/clinician-of-the-future-education-edition?utm_source=banner&utm_medium=dg&utm_campaign=cotf&utm_content=srpt#1ackowms1mu2erhf3vhv7u
4. Projected physician shortage: https://www.aamc.org/news/press-releases/new-aamc-report-shows-continuing-projected-physician-shortage
5. Survey of burnout in physicians: https://www.mayoclinicproceedings.org/article/S0025-6196(22)00515-8/fulltext#%20

Essay 28

1. A physician's account of "quiet firing": https://www.kevinmd.com/2024/08/quiet-firing-in-medicine-my-journey-from-burnout-to-freedom.html
2. Medical director demographics and statistics: https://www.zippia.com/medical-director-jobs/demographics/

Essay 31

1. Treatment-resistant depression: https://www.ncbi.nlm.nih.gov/pmc/articles/PMC10503923/
2. "Swedish" study: https://psychiatryonline.org/doi/10.1176/appi.ajp.20230353

Essay 36

1. Pete Townshend quote: https://www.songfacts.com/facts/pete-townshend/cant-outrun-the-truth

Essay 37

1. Impact of "Dobbs" on reproductive health: https://www.guttmacher.org/2024/05/clear-and-growing-evidence-dobbs-harming-reproductive-health-and-freedom; and https://www.ansirh.org/research/research/care-post-roe-how-post-roe-laws-are-obstructing-clinical-care

Essay 38

1. The delayed return of Native remains: https://www.propublica.org/series/the-repatriation-project
2. The mentally ill in prisons: https://www.prisonpolicy.org/research/mental_health/
3. New York Times article: https://www.nytimes.com/2024/09/01/business/acadia-psychiatric-patients-trapped.html?smid=nytcore-ios-share&referringSource=articleShare&sgrp=c-cb&ngrp=ctr&pvid=C6140B9E-88DA-49C7-A18F-DA8872B88BF6

Essay 39

1. Meredith Vieira and Dr. Ronald Schouten quotes: https://archive.vanityfair.com/article/2016/2/man-of-her-dreams
2. Meeks quote/report: https://www.columbusmonthly.com/story/lifestyle/features/2022/03/29/michael-swango-serial-killer-dick-harp-jenniefer-harp-yanka/7138639001/

Essay 40

1. No Surprises Act: https://www.cms.gov/newsroom/fact-sheets/no-surprises-understand-your-rights-against-surprise-medical-bills

Essay 43

1. The "ultimate betrayal": https://www.theguardian.com/music/2023/nov/30/the-ultimate-betrayal-more-details-emerge-in-hall-oates-lawsuit

Essay 44

1. Kristin Neff/self-compassion article: https://self-compassion.org/wp-content/uploads/publications/SCtheoryarticle.pdf

Essay 46

1. Negative impact of unwell physicians: https://www.sciencedirect.com/science/article/pii/S0140673609614240?dgcid=api_sd_search-api-endpoint

Essay 47

1. "A Trickle-Down Model of Abusive Supervision": https://onlinelibrary.wiley.com/doi/abs/10.1111/j.1744-6570.2012.01246.x
2. UVA faculty letter of no-confidence: https://www.cavalierdaily.com/article/2024/09/uva-health-faculty-demand-removal-of-health-system-ceo-school-of-medicine-dean

Essay 49

1. 2023 Main Residency Match Results: https://www.nrmp.org/wp-content/uploads/2023/03/2023-Advance-Data-Tables-FINAL.pdf
2. *BMC Medical Education* article: https://bmcmededuc.biomedcentral.com/articles/10.1186/s12909-023-04598-2
3. *Science* article: https://www.science.org/doi/10.1126/science.847460
4. Rochester-Temple drug discovery partnership: https://www.urmc.rochester.edu/news/story/urmc-and-temple-university-announce-drug-discovery-partnership

Essay 50

1. *The Wall Street Journal* article: https://www.wsj.com/personal-finance/caregiving-aging-at-home-retirement-103520c7

2. “The Compression of Morbidity”: https://www.ncbi.nlm.nih.gov/pmc/articles/PMC2690269/
3. “Is There Compression of Morbidity?”: https://www.ncbi.nlm.nih.gov/pmc/articles/PMC3001754/

Essay 51

1. CNBC survey: https://www.cnbc.com/2024/09/06/survey-how-many-americans-plan-to-work-in-retirement.html?utm_campaign=trueanthem&utm_medium=social&utm_source=linkedin%7Cmakeit

www.ingramcontent.com/pod-product-compliance
Lightning Source LLC
Chambersburg PA
CBHW070619220526
45466CB00001B/56

* 9 7 8 1 6 6 3 2 6 7 6 8 9 *